EVALUATION AND MANAGEMENT OF HOSPITAL INFECTIONS

NEW PERSPECTIVES IN CLINICAL MICROBIOLOGY 5

Other volumes in this series:

1. Brumfitt W, ed Hamilton-Miller JMT, ass. ed: New perspectives in clinical microbiology. 1978. ISBN 90-247-2074-5
2. Tyrrell DAJ, ed: Aspects of slow and persistent virus infections. 1979. ISBN 90-247-2281-0
3. Brumfitt W, Curcio L, Silvestri L, eds: Combined antimicrobial therapy. 1979. ISBN 90-247-2280-2
4. van Furth R, ed: Developments in antibiotic treatment of respiratory infections. 1981. ISBN 90-247-2493-7.

Series ISBN 90-247-2329-9

EVALUATION AND MANAGEMENT OF HOSPITAL INFECTIONS

edited by

RALPH VAN FURTH

Department of Infectious Diseases
University Hospital, Leiden
The Netherlands

1982

MARTINUS NIJHOFF PUBLISHERS
THE HAGUE / BOSTON / LONDON

Distributors:

for the United States and Canada

Kluwer Boston, Inc.
190 Old Derby Street
Hingham, MA 02043
USA

for all other countries

Kluwer Academic Publishers Group
Distribution Center
P.O. Box 322
3300 AH Dordrecht
The Netherlands

Library of Congress Cataloging in Publication Data CIP

Main entry under title:

Evaluation and management of hospital infections.

(New perspectives in clinical microbiology ; v. 5)
1. Nosocomial infections--Prevention--Congresses.
2. Nosocomial infections--Congresses. 3. Hospitals
--Hygiene--Congresses. I. Furth, Ralph van.
II. Series. [DNLM: 1. Cross infection--Congresses.
2. Drug resistance--Congresses. W1 NE484C
v.5 / WX 167 E92 1982]
RA969.E9 1982 616'.047 82-14490
ISBN 90-247-2754-5
ISBN 90-247-2760-X (pbk.)

ISBN 90-247-2754-5 (this volume)
ISBN 90-247-2760-X (paper)
ISBN 90-247-2329-9 (series)

PRINTED IN THE NETHERLANDS

The organization of this symposium held at Noordwijkerhout, The Netherlands, March 26-27, 1982, and the publication of the proceedings have been made possible by financial support from Bristol Myers BV. The help of Ms J. A. Kaat, Mrs. H. Muhren, and Ms I. Seeger-Wolf in preparing the manuscripts and discussions for publication is gratefully acknowledged.

CONTENTS

LIST OF CONTRIBUTORS XI

1. Introduction
R. van Furth 1

2. Evaluation of antimicrobial resistance
D.R. Schaberg 7

3. Plasmid typing as an epidemiological tool
B. van Klingeren 13

Discussion 17

4. Clinical implications of acquired antimicrobial resistance
I. Phillips 20

5. Antibiotic resistance in various municipalities in The Netherlands
M.F. Michel 30

Discussion 34

6. Antibiotic prescribing in a general hospital
F. Moss 37

7. Insights into antibacterial pharmacotherapy and measures leading to control of drug use
C.W.R. Phaf 49

Discussion 56

8. Antimicrobial resistance in hospital: New trends and control
R.A. Weinstein 58

9. Computer monitoring of drug resistance in the hospital
R.P. Mouton 75

Discussion 82

10. Occurrence of infections and antibiotic prophylaxis in non-surgical patients
P.J. van den Broek and W.E. Fibbe 85

11. Implications and consequences of antimicrobial therapy for the development and transfer of resistance
D. van der Waaij 119

Discussion 128

12. Don't touch the blade: Control of surgical sepsis
O.M. Lidwell 131

13. Comments on the occurrence and prophylaxis of surgical infections
R.K.J. Koumans 151

Discussion 155

14. Nosocomial infections in compromised hosts
L.S. Young 160

15. Antibiotic strategy in myelocompromised patients
J.W.M. van der Meer, W.E. Fibbe and
P.J. van den Broek 173

Discussion 178

16. Bacterial infection in the critically-ill neonate
D.A. Goldmann 180

17. Nosocomial infections in the neonatal intensive
care unit
J.J. Roord, R.Ch. Senders and A. Fleer 200

Discussion 206

18. Infection in the renal transplant patient
N.E. Tolkhoff-Rubin and R.H. Rubin 209

19. Factors contributing to an increased infection rate
after kidney transplantation
J.P. van Hooff and P.J. van den Broek 222

Discussion 226

20. Cost-benefit aspects of surveillance of hospital
infections
R.W. Haley 230

21. Comments on issues in studying the cost-benefit
of hospital infection surveillance and control
programs
J.I. Hudson 244

Discussion 249

22. Future trends in nosocomial infections:
Understanding selectivity and specificity in
microbial opportunism
G.G. Jackson 251

LIST OF CONTRIBUTORS

Broek van der, P.J., Afdeling Infectieziekten, Academisch Ziekenhuis, Rijnsburgerweg 10, 2333 AA Leiden, The Netherlands

Furth van, R., Afdeling Infectieziekten, Academisch Ziekenhuis, Rijnsburgerweg 10, 2333 AA Leiden, The Netherlands

Goldmann, D.A., Division of Infectious Diseases, The Children's Hospital, Medical Center, 3000 Longwood Avenue, Boston, MA 02115, U.S.A.

Haley, R.W., Hospital Infections Program, Center for Infectious Diseases, Centers for Disease Control, Atlanta, GA 30333, U.S.A.

Hooff van, J.P., Afdeling Nierziekten, Ziekenhuis St. Annadal, Postbus 1918, 6201 BX Maastricht, The Netherlands

Hudson, J.I., Centraal Begeleidingsorgaan voor de Intercollegiale Toetsing, Beneluxlaan 39, 3526 KK Utrecht, The Netherlands

Jackson, G.G., Section of Infectious Diseases, Department of Medicine, Abraham Lincoln School of Medicine, University of Illinois College of Medicine, P.O. Box 6998, Chicago, IL 60680, U.S.A.

Klingeren van, B., Rijksinstituut voor de Volksgezondheid, Postbus 1, 3720 BA Bilthoven, The Netherlands

Koumans, R.K.J., Afdeling Chirurgie, Westeinde Ziekenhuis, Lijnbaan 32, 2512 VA The Hague, The Netherlands

Lidwell, O.M., M.R.C. Common Cold Unit, Harvard Hospital, Coombe Road, Salisbury, Wilts SP2 8BW, England

Meer van der, J.W.M., Afdeling Infectieziekten, Academisch Ziekenhuis, Rijnsburgerweg 10, 2333 AA Leiden, The Netherlands

Michel, M.F., Afdeling Bacteriologie, Academisch Ziekenhuis - Dijkzigt, Dr. Molewaterplein 40, 3015 GD Rotterdam, The Netherlands

Moss, F., Whittington Hospital, Highgate Wing, Highgate Hill, London N19 5NF, England

Mouton, R.P., Afdeling Medische Microbiologie, Academisch Ziekenhuis, Rijnsburgerweg 10, 2333 AA Leiden, The Netherlands

Phaf, C.W.R., Ziekenhuis Apotheek, Ziekenhuis St. Annadal, Postbus 1918, 6201 BX Maastricht, The Netherlands

Phillips, I., Department of Microbiology, St. Thomas' Hospital, Medical School, London SE1 7EH, England

Roord, J.J., Wilhelmina Kinderziekenhuis, Nieuwe Gracht 137, 3512 LK Utrecht, The Netherlands

Rubin, R.H., Infectious Diseases Unit, Massachusetts General Hospital, Boston, MA 02114, U.S.A.

Schaberg, D.R., University of Michigan, Medical Center, Division of Infectious Diseases, R 6022 Kresge II, 1405 East Ann Street, Ann Arbor, Michigan 48109, U.S.A.

Waaij van der, D., Laboratorium voor Medische Microbiologie, Academisch Ziekenhuis, Oostersingel 59, 9713 EZ Groningen, The Netherlands

Weinstein, R.A., Division of Infectious Diseases, Michael Reese Hospital and Medical Center, 29th Street and Ellis Avenue, Chicago, IL 60616, U.S.A.

Young, L.S., Division of Infectious Diseases, Department of Medicine, The Center for the Health Sciences University of California, Los Angeles, CA 90024, U.S.A.

INTRODUCTION

R. VAN FURTH

Infection is an inseparable part of communal life, and infections are more common and more severe in hospital communities because the sick are more easily infected than the healthy. However, even though progress in the medical sciences has meant that many more patients suffering from relatively severe diseases can be helped at present, the use of more sophisticated and complex treatment leads to impairment of the defence mechanisms in more patients than was the case ten to twenty years ago, and these patients are also more prone to develop an infection.

Two questions are particularly relevant in this context. 1) Under what conditions do hospital infections occur? Defects of host defence mechanisms are of great importance in this respect. Such defects can be due to the disease or to the treatment given to the patient. 2) Which of the host defence mechanisms can be affected by a stay in the hospital? Among the factors involved in the host defence against infections (Table I), a number are especially important in this respect. For instance, venepuncture, indwelling catheters, and surgery all cause a breach in the surface structures. Anaesthesia causes temporary impairment of mechanical factors. Vascularization may be defective -- especially in the aged and patients with diabetes mellitus -- and this may complicate the healing of wounds in the skin and mucous membranes after surgery. The nutritional state is extremely important, because wound healing may be disturbed in the obese and malnourished, and infections are difficult to control in patients with endocrine disorders. All kinds of chemotherapy and other forms of treatment may interfere with host defence mechanisms, and patients are particularly susceptible to infections when granulocytopenia is severe, i.e., fewer than 500 cells per mm^3.

Table I.

FACTORS INVOLVED IN THE HOST DEFENCE AGAINST INFECTIONS

Surface structures	Horny layer of skin Mucosal epithelia
Surface secretions	Fatty acids and lactic acid of skin secretions Gastric acid
Mechanical factors	Ciliary movement Intestinal motility
Non-specific humoral factors	Lysozyme Lactoferrin Transferrin Complement
Specific humoral factors (immunoglobulins)	Antibodies
Cells	Polymorphonuclear leucocytes Mononuclear phagocytes (macrophages and monocytes) Lymphocytes
Vascularization	
Age	
Nutritional state	

Infections can be caused by micro-organisms either already carried by the patient himself (endogenous flora) or originating from another patient or personnel or inaminate objects (exogenous flora). When infections of the latter type occur in a hospital, they are called hospital-acquired infections to distinguish them from the community-acquired infections.

An important point with respect to hospital infections is the possibility of patients becoming colonized with new micro-organisms while in the hospital. Such newly acquired bacteria may have a pattern of antibiotic sensitivity differing from that of the patient's endogenous bacteria, and may even be multi-resistant. Colonization is unquestionably promoted by treatment of patients with antimicrobial drugs used for either therapeutic or long-term prophylactic purposes. The main problem associated with the colonization of patients by (multi-)resistant bacteria in the hospital is that it may lead to the failure of standard regimens for routine antibiotic prophylaxis in surgery and the initial treatment of infections.

In view of the many risks to which patients are exposed during a stay in a hospital it would be interesting to know the true incidence of hospital-acquired infections, but such information is scarce. It may be assumed that in developed countries 5% of all admitted patients will acquire an infection during hospitalization; the rate varies among the wards, the highest usually being reported for surgical wards, followed by the medical and obstetrical-gynaecological wards. The rate is higher for very young infants and older people than for the other age groups. According to the summarized data from eight studies, given in Table II, the number of hospital-acquired infections showed no marked changes between 1964 and 1975 (1).

Table II.

INFECTIONS IN HOSPITAL PATIENTS*

Infections	Community-acquired	Hospital-acquired	All infections
Urinary	15	30	22
Upper respiratory	6	3	5
Lower respiratory	32	17	25
Wound: minor	1	11	6
major	1	8	5
Skin	18	14	16
Female genital	4	4	4
Gastro-intestinal	3	1	2

* from reference 1

A survey of the prevalence of hospital infections in England and Wales yielded some very interesting data (1). For instance, the infections most frequently acquired in ahospital were urinary-tract infections (30% of all infections), and these were found almost twice as often in females as in males. The results also showed that 9% of all patients had been catheterized, that 21% of the catheterized and 3% of the non-catheterized patients developed a urinary-tract infection, and that among the infected patients, 41% had been catheterized. These figures raise the question whether catheterization is properly performed; it seems highly probable that a proportion of these hospital-acquired infections can be prevented. Another interesting finding made in this prevalence study is that 78% of the infected non-catheterized patients, 60% of the infected catheterized patients, and 31% of the non-infected catheterized patients were treated with antimicrobial drugs. It is extremely doubtful that this treatment was necessary in the last two of these groups of patients. Among the other localizations the respiratory tract took the lead, such infections accounting for about 30% of the cases; in about 5% of them the upper respiratory tract was involved and in about 25% the lower respiratory tract. However, most of the latter infections (16%) were community acquired, which means that the patient had already had the infection before admission. In this survey, furthermore, about 5% of all wounds were infected, which is only slightly lower than the percentage found in other surveys.

These examples give an impression of the occurrence of hospital-acquired infections, which are still a serious problem. It is therefore very important to be aware of the risks a patient runs on being admitted to a hospital. Familiarity with the current state of affairs seems to produce oblivion: despite the regular presence of infection in the wards, the hospital's doctors and nurses frequently deny its existence, and acknowledge it only in the more exceptional circumstances of an outbreak. This situation often leads to overreaction when such events overtake the hospital staff, and this in turn sometimes leads them to take measures based not on careful consideration or proven facts but on belief.

The consequences of hospital-acquired infections for the patient are pain and misery, temporarily impaired functions, and perhaps even death. But these infections also involve an increased burden of extra expenditure for treatment and a longer stay in the hospital. In a recent study the extra costs were calculated of longer nursing in a hospital because of infection after colon surgery if short-term prophylaxis is not applied. If we assume for The Netherlands that 32,000 colon operations are performed a year (Centrum voor Informatie Verwerking Nederlandse Ziekenhuizen), and that the rate of infections amounts to 10%, the duration of hospitalization is increased by about 13 days (2), and one day in a hospital costs 600 Dutch guilders, we arrive at a total figure of about 25 million guilders extra hospital costs per year, not including the costs of the drugs, bandages, etc.

During the past year, interest in the control of hospital infections has increased. We must, however, define the conditions to be considered mandatory for reduction of the number infections acquired in the hospital, for example:

Awareness of endemic hospital-acquired infections.

Availability of quantitative information about endemic hospital infections.

Identification of areas in the hospital where infections are more likely to occur.

Rapid recognition of an outbreak of infections.

Awareness of the greater susceptibility of some categories of patients to infection by certain micro-organisms.

Awareness that some kinds of surgical or drug treatment make patients more susceptible to infections.

Availability of adequate regimes for prophylaxis with respect to infections.

Maintenance of a restricted antibiotic policy throughout the hospital.

Continous education and practical instruction for the entire staff of the hospital.

Implementation of the regimens for aseptic techniques by infection-control personnel.

Awareness of the cost-benefit relationship in infection control.

All these measures can contribute to the improvement of the well-being of patients, but it is of great importance to establish priorities. Not all of the necessary conditions can be adequately maintained at all times in all hospitals, because sufficient funds and personnel are lacking. Although it must be realized that not all infections are preventable, we must continue to make every possible effort to decrease the incidence of hospital-acquired infections.

At present, most hospitals have an Infection Committee or at least an infection-control nurse. In the Leiden University Hospital an infection committee was instituted in 1960, when Staphylococcus aureus infections became an urgent problem in hospitals throughout the world. Since this committee was established, the field it covers has been repeatedly enlarged, and at present this hospital employs three infection-control nurses and two technicians specialized in hospital epidemiology.

The impulse for this symposium arose from the increasing interest in the problem of hospital infections in The Netherlands.This problem must be considered urgent, not only because of the effects on the patients but also because of the financial repercussions. The symposium was organized to provide an opportunity for the disussion of various aspects of the occurrence and prevention of these infections.

REFERENCES

1. Report on the National Survey of Infection in Hospitals, 1980, 1981. J. Hosp. Inf. 2 (suppl).
2. Ulrich C. 1981. Short term systemic antibiotic prophylaxis in colorectal surgery. Thesis, Leiden University.

EVALUATION OF ANTIMICROBIAL RESISTANCE

D.R. SCHABERG

Resistance to antimicrobial agents in nosocomial pathogens profoundly affects many individuals involved in the complex process of delivering care to seriously ill, hospitalized patients. The greatest concern occurs when resistance to "first-choice" agents is seen, such as aminoglycoside resistance in gram-negative bacilli or Streptococcus faecalis, and methicillin resistance in S. aureus. The exchange of information between microbiologist, clinician, and epidemiologist takes on added significance as individuals usually less actively aware of nosocomial infection heighten their attention because of infection resistant to usual therapy.

Investigation of outbreaks of resistant organisms usually involves attempts to determine the origin of the resistant strains, their reservoir within the hospital, mode of transmission, and alternative therapeutic agents ; all useful in designing control measures. Other discussions will deal with various strategies for control of resistant organisms.

ROLE OF SURVEILLANCE

The detection and determination of the potential of a problem with resistant nosocomial infection is best made against background surveillance data. Ongoing tabulation of sensitivity testing results carried out in the clinical microbiology laboratory allows early detection of isolates with unusual antimicrobial susceptibilities. The choice of antimicrobial agents to serve as "flags" often depends on species and recent experience of the individual hospital with resistant strains. For example, where once resistance to gentamicin and tobramycin was rare at the University of Michigan Medical Center, now 6 % of Enterobacteriaeceae are resistant. Available resources do not allow detailed investigation of all gentamicin resistant infections. However, amikacin resistance remains uncommon and when resistant isolates are recognized, the organisms are retained for further study while the clinical and epidemiologic circumstances of the infection are investigated. In a similar manner, methicillin resistance triggers additional investigation in S. aureus isolates. In other words, the unusual is most easily recognized when in depth information about the usual is available.

CLONAL DISSEMINATION

When a problem with nosocomial infection resistant to antimicrobials is recognized, one important question to answer is whether the problem involves spread of a single strain or whether multiple strains are involved. Several techniques are useful in determining strain identity and provide varying levels of certainty that two isolates are, in fact, the same strain (1). The most widely used and available techniques are those that result from the original evaluation of an isolate in the clinical laboratory including the speciation of the isolate and its antimicrobial susceptibility. Genus and species identification is usually not sufficient, but on occasion, an unusual biochemical profile or "biotype" may allow presumptive evidence for identity between isolates. Likewise, antimicrobial susceptibility patterns or antibiograms also can be used to provide information on whether resistant isolates are the same. Additional clues to strain identity can be obtained by not only examining the "S" and "R" pattern of suspected identical isolates but by also examining the actual zone of inhibition determined by Kirby-Bauer testing or actual MIC by broth or agar dilution. Unfortunately, many nosocomial pathogens provide too little variability in biotype or antibiogram to allow accurate determination of the identical nature of isolates.

Additional typing information can be obtained from referral centers and is usually dependent upon the species to be examined. Serotyping, phage typing, bacteriocin production, and bacteriocin susceptibility can be useful depending on the organism. An additional procedure which has provided information useful for typing isolates has been analysis of the total plasmid content of bacterial cells by agarose gel electrophoresis (AGE) (3). Recent technical advances now allow such analyses to be completed within two days of isolation of an organism in pure culture (2). We have found the information generated by AGE most important in organisms such as Citrobacter species, Enterobacter, and non-aeruginosa Pseudomonas species where other typing systems are not available. It should be noted, however, that all typing systems have liabilities and the information provided is most useful when coupled with other epidemiologic information.

PLASMID DISSEMINATION

In addition to clonal dissemination, which often leads to descriptions such as "our resistant Serratia", it is now clear that intergeneric R-plasmid exchange can and has contributed to problems encountered with resistant pathogens in a number of hospitals (5). Common features of all these reports has been their occurence in large referral hospitals, involvement of special care units, and simultaneous acquisition by the recipient of the "epidemic" R-plasmid of resistance to gentamicin and/or tobramycin and carbenicillin.

The evaluation of these outbreaks was facilitated by applying techniques popularized by Falkow and co-workers (3,6). Comparison of patterns of resistance is coupled with observation of the ability of the natural isolates to transfer similar resistances into reference host strains. Strains from a single environment transferring similar resistances are then analyzed along with their transconjugants for total plasmid content by AGE. Plasmids encoding similar resistances and of approximately the same size can be further explored for identity by endonuclease restriction analysis which provides a characteristic DNA fragment pattern (figure 1). Demonstration of identical size plasmids encoding for identical resistances with identical restriction endonuclease fragment patterns in multiple genera in the same hospital strongly supports intergeneric R-plasmid exchange within the hospital environment. How important R-plasmid exchange is in the overall picture of resistance remains unclear but certainly in the large hospital in special care areas where selective pressure of therapy is greatest this mechanism can and does operate.

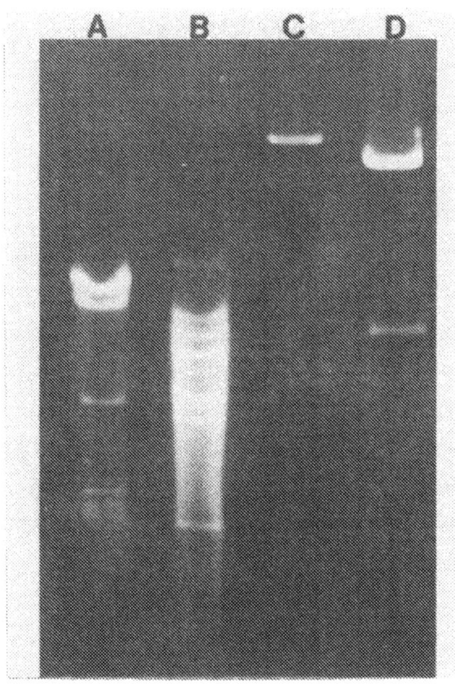

FIGURE 1. Agarose gel electrophoresis of plasmid DNA from two Klebsiella pneumoniae isolates originally felt to be related based on antimicrobial susceptibility. Plasmid profiles of each isolate are shown in C and D showing a single large plasmid in C and a different pattern in D. The large plasmids were transferred to E.coli and plasmid DNA obtained and digested with Eco R-1 shown in A and B confirming their differences.

TRANSPOSITION

Until recently, little insight was available into how multiple antimicrobial resistances come to reside on a single R-plasmid. It is now clear that the movement of resistance genes from one replicon to another via transposition can play an important role in the dissemination of resistance. The studies of Rubens and co-workers (4) clearly show how this process can work in the hospital environment. They showed that a gentamicin transposon originally present on a small, nonconjugative plasmid "hopped" onto a preexisting conjugative element and then was efficiently spread to other genera. Techniques for evaluating this process remain cumbersome and exclusively in the research laboratory. However, from the research studies completed so far, this mechanism is obviously important in the process of constructing R-plasmids carrying multiple resistances.

Table 1.
TECHNIQUES FOR EVALUATING ANTIMICROBIAL RESISTANCE

Level of genetic organization for resistance	Hospital based information for assessment	Referral or research assessment
Clonal dissemination of a strain	Antibiogram, biotyping	Serotyping, bacteriocin typing, phage typing, plasmid profile
Plasmid dissemination	"Expanded" antibiogram	Plasmid transfer, incompatability testing, plasmid profiles
Transposition	None	Analysis for transposition

CONCLUSIONS

The evolution of antimicrobial resistance is a complex process and involves multiple factors. In the hospital, antimicrobial therapy and other factors create an environment selecting for accelerated evolution of resistant strains. Evaluation of these resistant strains is aided by an awareness of the three levels of genetic organization which can be important when problems with antimicrobial resistance are encountered.

REFERENCES

1. Aber, R.C., Mackel, D.C. 1981. Epidemiologic typing of nosocomial microorganisms. Am. J. Med. 70 : 899.
2. Kado, C.I., Liu, S.T. 1981. Rapid procedure for detection and isolation of large and small plasmids. J. Bacteriol. 145 : 1365.
3. Meyers, J.A., Sanchez, D., Elwell, L.P., Falkow, S. 1976. Simple agarose gel electrophoretic method for the identification and characterization of plasmid deoxyribonucleic acid. J. Bacteriol. 127 : 1529.
4. Rubens, C.E., McNeill, W.F., Farrar, W.E. 1979. Evolution of transposable deoxyribonucleid-acid sequences. J. Bacteriol. 140 : 713.
5. Schaberg, D.R., Rubens, C.E., Alford, R.H., Farrar, W.E., Schaffner, W., McGee, Z.A. 1981. Evolution of antimicrobial resistance and nosocomial infection : Lessons from the Vanderbilt experience. Am. J. Med. 70 : 445.
6. Tompkins, L.S., Plorde, J.J., Falkow, S. 1980. Molecular analysis of R-factors from multi-resistant nosocomial isolates. J. Infect. Dis. 141 : 625.

PLASMID TYPING AS AN EPIDEMIOLOGICAL TOOL

B. VAN KLINGEREN

In National Institute of Public Health, studies on bacterial resistance to antibiotics started some twenty years ago with the surveillance of resistance in Salmonella. More recently, coordination of the surveillance of penicillinase-producing gonococci in The Netherlands was undertaken in our Institute. On a smaller scale, the incidence of resistance to clinically important antibiotics is surveilled in Ps. aeruginosa and H. influenzae. In all of these species resistance is predominantly plasmid mediated. So plasmid typing may provide an important epidemiological parameter.

Plasmid identification based on agarose gel electrophoresis (AGE) was introduced in our institute some years ago by Dr. J.D.A. van Embden. The early procedures for plasmid DNA isolation were rather time consuming and not very suitable for the routine screening of large numbers of bacterial strains. Recently, we adopted the technique described by Kado and Liu (1) for routine plasmid typing in penicillinase-producing strains of N. gonorrhoeae (PPNG). With this technique, which can also be used to analyse Gram-negative rods, 20 to 30 strains can be examined within a few hours. Fig. 1 shows the four plasmid patterns hitherto observed in PPNG strains, i.e., the "African" type 3.3 megadalton (Md) and the "Asian" type 4.5 Md plasmids, without or together with the 24 Md transfer plasmid (2). Since the incidence of these patterns differs from town to town and can change rapidly, information about the shifts or plasmid patterns may contribute to an understanding of the epidemiology of the strains harbouring them.

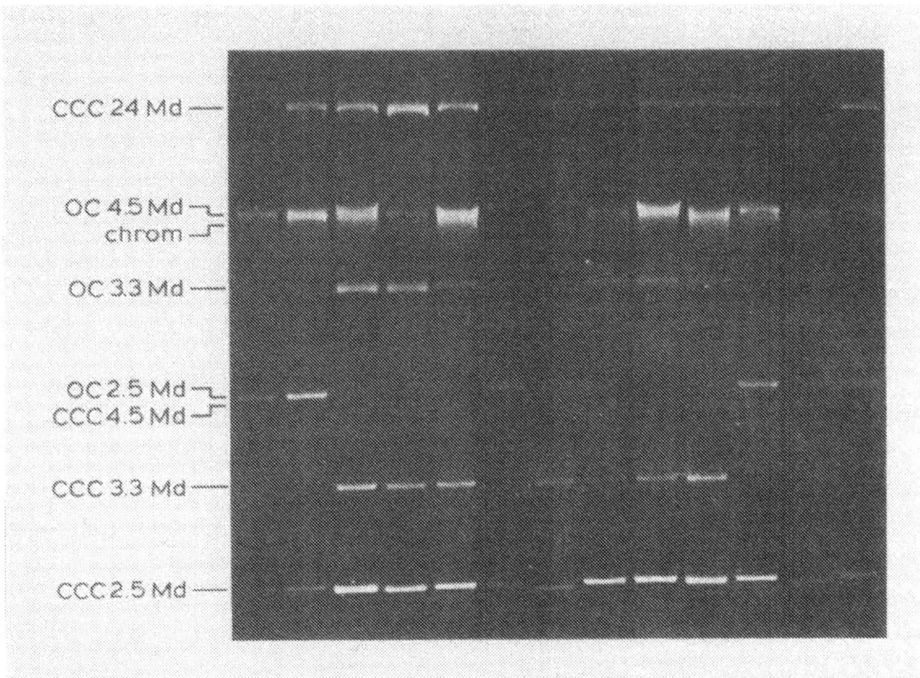

Fig. 1. Plasmid patterns in β-lactamase-producing strains of Neisseria gonorrhoeae.

Agarose gel electrophoresis of plasmid DNA is particularly useful for bacterial species for which biotyping, serotyping, or phage typing is lacking or insufficient, for example Klebsiella, Serratia, and Pseudomonas species. For these organisms this technique has already proven to be very useful to detect outbreaks of nosocomial infections (3-5). Fig. 2 illustrates this for Ps. aeruginosa. We examined strains from four hospitals. "A" pertains to an outbreak of gentamicin- and carbenicillin-resistant strains in hospital A. More than 20 patients acquired an infection caused by this strain. Thirteen isolates were analysed and the plasmid DNA in all of these strains appeared to be identical. As a reference, use was made of a Salm. java strain carrying plasmids in the range of 25 to 82 Md. "B" refers to a

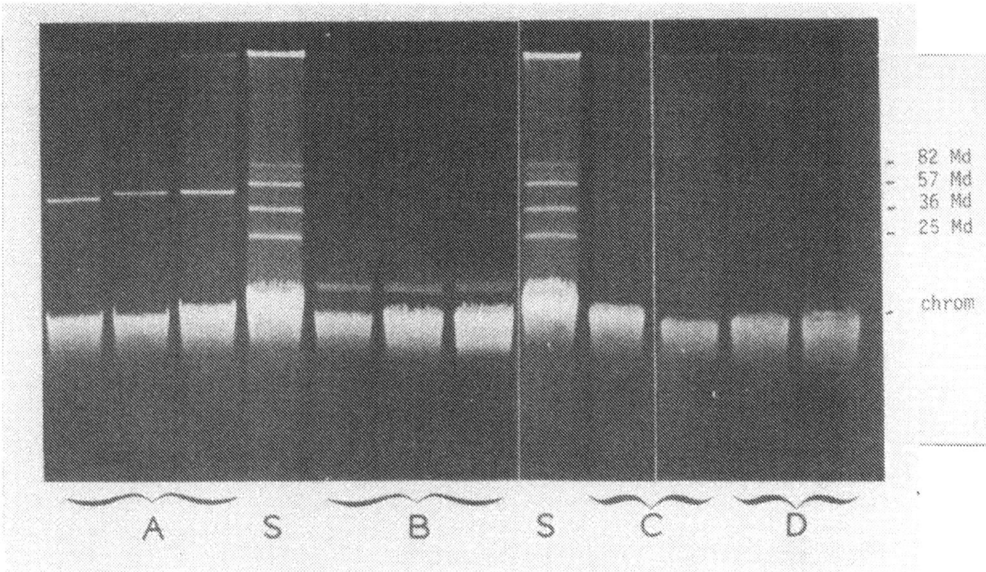

Fig. 2. Plasmids in Pseudomonas aeruginosa. A, B, C, and D: patient clusters in different hospitals. S: reference of strain of Salm. java harbouring several plasmids with characterized molecular weights.

cluster of strains from another hospital. These strains were resistant to gentamicin but susceptable to carbenicillin. In strains from hospitals C and D with different resistance patterns, no plasmids were found. This four-hospital example supports the view that agarose gel electrophoresis of plasmid DNA offers -- particularly when the easy and rapid method described by Kado and Liu is used -- a simple tool for obtaining a better understanding of the epidemiology of hospital infections and the intergeneric transfer of resistance determinants in the hospital environment.

There is another area where agarose gel electrophoresis may be helpful: with the exception of Salmonella, most observations indicate that selective pressure due to the use of antibiotics, in human medical practice is the major cause of the spread of multiple resistant strains in infections in man. However, the importance for human medical practice of the build up of plasmids in the veterinary field due to veterinary use of antibiotics, is controversial. For a better understanding of the possible promiscuity of "human" and "veterinary" plasmids, the agarose gel electrophoresis technique may prove to be very useful.

REFERENCES

1. Kado, C.I., Liu, S.T. 1981. Rapid procedure for detection and isolation of large and small plasmids. J. Bacteriol. 145: 1365.
2. Embden van, J.D.A., Klingeren van, B., Dessens-Kroon, M., Wijngaarden van, L.J. 1981. Emergence in The Netherlands of penicillinase-producing gonococci carrying "Africa" plasmid in combination with transfer plasmid. Lancet i: 938.
3. Schaberg, D.R., Rubens, C.E., Alford, R.H. et al. 1981. Evolution of antimicrobial resistance and nosocomial infection. Am. J. Med. 70: 445.
4. Schaberg, D.R., Tompkins, L.S., Falkow, S. 1981. Use of agarose gel electrophoresis of plasmid deoxyribonucleic acid to fingerprint Gram-negative bacilli. J. Clin. Microb. 13: 1105.
5. Olexy, V.M., Macha, D.K., Bird, T.J. et al. 1982. An R plasmid of Serratia marcescens transferable to Pseudomonas aeruginosa. Chemotherapy 28: 6.

DISCUSSION EDITED BY B. VAN KLINGEREN

van der Waay: Is bacterial conjugation possible in the undisturbed gastro-intestinal flora? What is your opinion of selective decontamination of patients at risk to prevent overgrowth of resistant organisms during antimicrobial therapy and to eliminate bacteria that can become receptors for plasmids?

Schaberg: I do not think that the kind of gene exchange we have been discussing here takes place in the gastro-intestinal tract; it occurs in the urinary tract and in urine-collection devices. We observed transfer of large molecular weight plasmids from Serratia to E. coli within about 20 minutes after inoculating these strains in urine. I think that in the hospital environment there is a variety of aqueous reservoirs containing sufficient amounts of nutrients to allow transfer of resistance determinants, for instance urine bags and dialysis fluid. Control of these resevoirs and other control measures are more important and simpler than selective decontamination. Without doing terrible things to the gastro-intestinal flora, it is almost impossible to get strains like the ones discussed to exchange genetic information in the gastro-intestinal tract. Moreover, many of the organisms involved in the observed outbreaks, for instance Serratia and Providentia, do not colonize the gastro-intestinal tract very well. On theoretical grounds one might expect gene exchange to occur in neonates or in someone whose gastro-intestinal flora is disturbed by large amounts of antimicrobials. Under those circumstances there might be a role for selective decontamination using drugs to which resistance has never been found in plasmids -- in particular polymyxins and nalidixic acid

-- to eliminate plasmid-bearing bacteria from the urinary tract and the gastro-intestinal tract.

Phillips: I confirm the importance of the urinary tract in the clinical context. In patients with several species and genera of bacteria carrying the same plasmid, the trail has always led back to the urinary tract. In those patients, who usually have bladder difficulties, you may find four or five different organisms and conjugation in the urine. These organisms get into the blood stream from time to time.

van Furth: In relation to cost-benefit evaluation, what is the size of the cluster of patients you start to investigate? From the computerized information about bacterial resistance and additional biotyping and phage typing in the University Hospital in Leiden it is obvious that different strains can be involved in clusters of three or four patients. I suppose that you have found many negative clusters too.

Schaberg: We too have found different strains when we were convinced we would find the same strain, but when one has three or more infections in the same ward or nursing unit caused by the same species or genus with the same susceptibility pattern, I myself want to know what is going on. It is not a magic number, but with three cases I begin to be suspicious.

Rubin: What is the relative importance for the nosocomial infection pattern of the three mechanisms you have described?

Schaberg: The overwhelming problem is clonal dissemination of individual strains. The role of plasmid exchange is probably underestimated, because in the hospital environment one is only interested in resistance to particular drugs. We get upset when we loose gentamicin but we do not care about ampicillin transfer, so I think exchange occurs more often than we recognize. I think transposition of genetic elements is very important in the construction of the large resistance plasmids.

van Klingeren: Do you have any views about the importance for human medical practice of the build up of plasmids in the veterinary field?

Schaberg: I think the veterinary use of drugs, especially antibiotics in animal feed, may perpetuate the maintenance of large resistance plasmids, since these plasmids not only carry resistance to determinants for gentamicin or carbenicillin but also for tetracycline, sulfonamides, and other agents. So tetracycline use is just as effective as gentamicin use in maintaining a gentamicin-resitant plasmid. In this way the use of antibiotics in veterinary practice may contribute to the problem of not only nosocomial infections but also in the Haemophilus, Salmonella, and other more traditional community infections.

Goldmann: I would like to illustrate the complexity of the situations that you are trying to analyse with the techniques you have mentioned. We had an outbreak of multiple-resistant Klebsiella in a paediatric surgical ward where a nurse was identified as a chronic carrier (on her hands) of Klebsiella. Nevertheless, different susceptibility patterns and different serotypes were found, so it was decided to carry out agarose gel electrophoresis. However, plasmids did not appear on the gels. So things can look very simple and be very complicated. I would also like to make another point about the reservoir of bacteria in the hospital as a place where genetic exchange may occur. Although in our hospital no catheters or large urine bags are used and urinary-tract infections are quite uncommon, plasmid exchange is observed, and I think this is almost certainly taking place in the gastro-intestinal tract.

Schaberg: Referring to my ealier comment, I think that neonates do not have all the complex flora that may be important in protecting against gene exchange. So it may be that gene exchange is common in the gut of neonates, but I think that in adults it is less important than other reservoirs.

CLINICAL IMPLICATIONS OF ACQUIRED ANTIMICROBIAL RESISTANCE

I. PHILLIPS

The assessment of the clinical significance of antibiotic resistance defined in the laboratory has seldom been based on the results of formal clinical trial, for the compelling reason that in most cases, such trials would be unethical. It is difficult to conceive that any doctor would agree to treat infection of any severity with an agent that could well fail when he can prescribe one that he knows will be effective. We must therefore be satisfied almost always with information gleaned from patients treated, with an "inappropriate" agent before the sensitivity of the pathogen has been determined.

However, this is not the only, or even the major difficulty. Any assessment is based on the assumptions that in-vitro resistance can be defined and determined and that the contribution of chemotherapy to patients' clinical course can be assessed. These assumptions require further analysis.

THE DEFINITION OF IN-VITRO RESISTANCE

The cornerstone of any in-vitro assessment of an antibiotic is the minimum inhibitory concentration (MIC) for the relevant pathogen. Although simple in concept - the lowest concentration of antibiotic that will inhibit the growth of the organism - it is complex in its determination. Firstly, it is subject to variability arising from differences in the artificial media in which it is determined, which may be more or less nutrient, variable in ionic content, and may possibly even contain inhibitors of antibacterial activity. Furthermore, its composition and thus its performance, may vary from batch to batch. A second set of variations arise from the particular bacterial culture used to inoculate the antibiotic-containing plates, the most important variable being the number of bacterial cells.

Fortunately many antibiotics and many organisms are little affected within a reasonable range of latitude, and results are surprisingly reproducible from time to time and from one laboratory to another. For others, comparisons are wellnigh impossible. Among antibacterials, sulphonamides pose considerable problems. We found that Bacteroides fragilis is usually sensitive to sulphonamides, which are potentiated by trimethoprim (1). In marked contrast, Rosenblatt and Stewart (2) in the USA concluded that the organism is usually resistant. When the American isolates were studied by our techniques they were found to be fully sensitive (3). Among organisms Haemophilus influenzae is a problem. Hamilton-Miller (4) has drawn attention to wide discrepancies in MICs of a variety of β -lactam antibiotics for H. influenzae and other organisms as determined by different laboratories, and to the need for uniformity of techniques.

The problem of standardisation applies equally to disc techniques, which are often preferred for routine use because of their supposed simplicity. Attempts to overcome irreproducibility have either been based on strict definition of technique or on the use of control organisms of known sensitivity. The Kirby-Bauer technique advocated by the National Committee for Clinical Laboratory Standards in the USA (5) prescribe a single medium, standardised discs and a fixed inoculum, and a rigidly-defined technique, while the Stokes' and comparative techniques used in the UK concentrate on a correct inoculum size and the use of control tests on the same or separate plates. Brown and Blowers (6) have reviewed the comparative performance of these techniques. As with MICs some disc tests are easy to control whil others are almost impossible, as revealed in the results of the British Quality Control scheme.

Although with rigorous control both MICs, and to a lesser extent disc tests, can be made reproducible and accurate, there remains the almost insuperable problem of the definition of resistance. Clearly one could expect a correlation between MIC and the likelihood of clinical success. If there is a bimodal distribution of MICs, when the two modes are widely separated, and when antibiotic concentrations available in infected tissues easily exceed the lower but fall well below the higher mode, this expectation is much more likely to be clearly demonstrable. If, however, MICs are continuously distributed, it merely becomes increasingly less probable that a patient will respond if he is infected with organisms with increasingly higher MICs. Decisions have to be made on a break point and on the use of such terms as "intermediate" and "moderate" resistance for the ill-defined zone. Much heat is generated in these discussions, but few conclusions are based on good experimental evidence.

Given reproducible results and agreed break points, the arguments then arise that disc tests and MICs represent the end-result of a complex series of events, which do not closely mimic the in-vivo situation. Attempts have been made to improve disc techniques, for example to assess the effects of β -lactamase induction (7). Other workers, including Greenwood & O'Grady (8) and Yourassowsky et al (9) have advocated the continuous monitoring of growth in liquid media to which antibiotics can be added in different concentrations and at different times. Such methods do amplify our knowledge of resistance but do not yield information of proven clinical relevance.

The recognition of the biochemical mechanisms of in-vitro resistance, such as the profusion of β -lactamases and aminoglycoside-modifying enzymes, has led to the hope that their detection might be used as the basis of the definition of resistance. It has become clear that quantitation of enzyme, permeability of the bacterial cell, and the kinetics of the enzyme-antibiotic interaction are also important, and that these factors and others account for the fact that the correlations between the presence of an enzyme and the MIC are often not good. When this is the case, it is not known which is more relevant to the clinical situation.

Clearly in-vitro resistance is not a simple, all-ornone phenomenon, nor is it clearly definable, and the assessment of the clinical relevance of antibiotic resistance must take all this into account.

RESPONSE TO CHEMOTHERAPY

The conclusion that the administration of an antibiotic has affected the clinical course of an infection is difficult surprisingly to many who have not tried to convince a desinterested observer. Its formal demonstration is easiest for an infection that runs a defined constant course and does not recover spontaneously either too quickly or erratically in the absence of chemotherapy. However, clinical trials are unethical when effective treatment is known to exist, and when the disease is severe or potentially fatal. Thus we cannot knowingly use antibiotics for which there is any indication of in-vitro resistance for the treatment of, for example, septicaemia or meningitis which might otherwise be useful models. Most of the infections in which it might be ethical to use a potentially ineffective drug are difficult to assess because of their variability, and this applies to most pyogenic infection in which the release of pus is often the single determinant of recovery. A similar difficulty of assessment also applies to patients whose recovery depends on immune mechanisms, for example patients with severe neutropenia whose white cells return. If it can be concluded that a patient's failure to recover is clearly linked to a failure of chemotherapy it is still necessary to exclude pharmacological factors, including failure of compliance, or of absorption, unusual distribution and excretion. It is seldom possible to demonstrate that active antibiotic has reached the "growing edge" of an infective lesion, although the detection of antibiotic in adequate amounts in blood and some body fluids may be used as an indirect indicator. The opposite anomaly of the patient who responds despite chemotherapy that appears inappropriate must also be explored. In-vitro resistance break points may well not apply if antibiotics are concentrated in urine or bile, for example.

In all anomalous responses, there is always the possibility that the microbiologist has chosen the wrong organism to investigate in the laboratory. For example, many Gram-negative bacilli isolated from sputum are merely colonising and not infecting the respiratory tract. Only with samples from a closed lesion can one be confident that one has the appropriate organisms, but in mixed infections there may still be difficulties in deciding which are the pathogens.

Neisseria gonorrhoeae

Gonorrhoea is one of the few diseases for which there is a completely convincing relationship between in-vitro resistance and response to chemotherapy. Gonococcal urethritis in males produces obvious symptoms and signs which continue at least in the short term until the patient is effectively treated. Samples for microbiological investigation are easy to obtain and results easy to interpret. In addition there are large numbers of patients, whose only failing is that of not returning for assessment when they are cured. The gonococcus has a variety of resistance mechanisms including high level and easily recognised resistance to streptomycin and spectinomycin, the production of a single well-characterised β -lactamase, and resistance based on impermeability to a variety of antibiotics including β -lactams. Finally gonorrhoea is a disease that is not massively overtreated as short-course or even single-dose treatment is preferred. Given these almost ideal circumstances it is reassuring to those who believe in the relevance of in-vitro test to find the convincing correlations.

Resistance to streptomycin is common, and although it has not been assessed for many years, results in an almost total failure of response to the drug. Spectinomycin resistance is rare but it too results in clinical failure (10). Although MICs for β -lactamase-producing gonococci range widely depending on inoculum, the correlation is between MICs for large inocula, or alternatively and more simply, the demonstration of the enzyme, and clinical failure, which approaches 100 % for these strains. On this evidence the correlation between high level resistance or β -lactamse production and clinical results is totally convincing.

Resistance to β -lactams other than via β -lactamase is more complex. Permeability to a variety of antibiotics is determined in a cumulative manner by a number of genetic mutations, and thus resistance to unrelated agents is uniquely linked. Fully sensitive organisms respond to a wide variety of β -lactams, and benzyl penicillin is among the most active. Moderately resistant organisms with benzyl penicillin MICs above 0.1 mg/l respond progressively less well to all β -lactams until for MICs above about 1 mg/l failure with normal single-dose regimens is the rule. Similar considerations apply to other antibacterials. Thus again, although the relationship is not all-or-none, there is a good correlation between MICs and clinical response.

Haemophilus influenzae

This organism has recently been found with resistance to ampicillin, some intrinsic, some associated with β -lactamase, and to chloramphenicol. Failures of therapy of meningitis with both agents have been reported, and clinical relevance cannot be doubted.

Streptococcus pneumoniae

The recently described intrinsic penicillin resistance in pneumococci in South Africa, although not of high level, has clearly resulted in failures of penicillin therapy in meningitis and failure of other agents for which resistance is associated with that of penicillin.

Salmonella typhi

Typhoid caused by organisms resistant to chloramphenicol and ampicillin fails to respond to therapy with these drugs.

Staphylococci

The commonest staphylococcal infections are self-limiting, and resolve with the release of pus - a somewhat unpredictable event. Conversely serious infections such as septicaemia often respond slowly to appropriate agents. It is again not surprising that β -lactamase production and the generalised β -lactam resistance usually referred to as methicillin resistance have been considered irrelevant by some, but I have been unable to find any trial to prove or disprove the point. One must suspect that if the variability of clinical course could be allowed for, relevance would be perceived. The relationship between inappropriate therapy and acquisition of a resistant organism during an epidemic is clearer (11).

Enterobacteria and Pseudomonas aeruginosa

Resistance among enterobacteria and Ps. aeruginosa is widely reported but because of true infections are vastly outnumbered by colonisations, especially of the respiratory tract, its significance is difficult to assess. Reports of failure to respond of severe infections, such as septicaemia, must be assessed against a background of underlying disease which is the most important determinant of response to chemotherapy. Patients with Gram-negative septicaemia complicating urinary tract instrumentation not uncommonly recover spontaneously while those with severe neutropenia often succumb despite appropriate chemotherapy, unless the neutropenia is reversed, in which case they often recover. Patients with an unreachable sump of infection often fail to respond even when their organisms are sensitive. Klastersky (12) has drawn attention to Gram-negative septicaemia, pneumonia and meningitis that behave in this way.

URINARY TRACT INFECTION

Assessment of the relevance of in-vitro sensitivity in urinary tract infections is complicated by two important factors, the first that antibiotics are usually considerably concentrated in urine and it is difficult in this context to define resistance in-vitro that will be clinically relevant, and the second is that the infection not infrequently disappears without chemotherapy. The poor correlation between resistance and response in this very common infection has contributed very considerably to doubts about the relevance of laboratory results which have sometimes been extrapolated to all infections.

PREVALENCE OF RESISTANCE

The overall effect of resistance depends on its prevalence. Many reports give no denominators and no prevalence rates, but give the impression that resistance is a common problem. Undoubtedly this is true in some places and at some times, and each microbiologist must determine the prevalence of resistance locally.

We have investigated resistance to carbenicillin and aminoglycosides in Ps. aeruginosa since 1976, when aminoglycoside resistance was first recognised in our hospital. A low plateau was rapidly reached and there has been little overall increase in recent years. Resistance to gentamycin is currently found in 6.1 % of isolates, to tobramycin in 2.1 %, to amikacin in 2.4 % and to carbenicillin in 7.6 %. Resistance to carbenicillin and gentamycin was found in only about 1 %.

The figures suggest that our problems with resistance in Ps. aerguinosa are not great but even they may not accurately reflect the problem. For example the rate of resistance in strains from the blood of patients with bacteremia may well differ.

We can prescribe gentamycin and carbenicillin with some confidence as initial therapy in patients with serious Ps. aeruginosa infections, unless the patient has acquired infection in certain wards of the hospital, in which case an isolate from another site or patient will often provide the necessary stimulus to use alternatives. This is important, since we wish to continue to use agents with which we are familiar rather than change to new ones that create new problems.

CONCLUSIONS

With care in-vitro resistance can be defined, and it seems wise to take note of the results of different methods of assessment in this definition. It will then be possible to determine its clinical relevance in a limited number of diseases, and extrapolation as well as limited, usually uncontrolled clinical observations will determine its likely relevance in others. If resistance becomes prevalent, changes in prescribing will inevitably follow, making further observations of the clinical relevance of in-vitro resistance impossible. The role of the microbiologist is to try to establish with his clinical colleagues, which in-vitro findings are important and which can safely be ignored. A failure to do this in the past has resulted in agnosticism among clinicians which can have unfortunate results if it is universally applied, especially when antibiotic dosages used are low and when infection is inaccessible or norma immunological mechanisms are impaired or overwhelmed.

REFERENCES

1. Phillips, I., Warren, C. 1974. The susceptibility of Bacteroides fragilis to trimethoprim and sulphamethoxazole. Lancet. 1 : 827.
2. Rosenblatt, J.E., Stewart, P.R. 1974. Lack of activity of sulphamethoxazole and trimethoprim against anaerobic bacteria. Antimicrob. Agents Chemother. 6 : 93.
3. Phillips, I., Warren, C. 1976. Activity of sulphamethoxazole and trimethoprim against Bacteroides fragilis. Antimicrob. Agents Chemother. 9 : 736.
4. Hamilton-Miller, J.M.T. 1977. Towards greater uniformity in sensitivity testing. J. Antimicrob. Chemother. 3 : 385.
5. Barry, A.L., Thornsberry, C. 1980. Susceptibility testing diffusion test procedures. In : Lennette E.H. (ed). Manual of Clinical Microbiology third edition. American Society for Microbiology, Washington.
6. Brown, D., Blowers, R. 1978. Methods of sensitivity testing and other semi-quantitative methods. In : D.S. Reeves, I. Phillips, J.D. Williams and R. Wise (eds). Laboratory Methods in Antimicrobial Chemotherapy. Churchill Livingstone, London.
7. Selwyn, S. 1980. The beta-lactam antibiotics : penicillins and cephalosporins in perspective. Hodder & Stoughton, London.
8. Greenwood, D., O'Grady, F. 1978. An in-vitro model of the urinary bladder. J. Antimicrob. Chemother. 4 : 113.

9. Yourassowsky, E., Van der Linden, M.P., Lismont, M.S., Crokaert, F. 1982. Early response of the growth curve to different beta-lactams concentration : a new approach for penicillin-binding proteins study. Proceedings of third International Symposium on Rapid Methods and Automation in Microbiology. American Society of Microbiology.
10. Centers for Disease Control 1981. Morbidity and Mortality Weekly Reports. 30 : 221.
11. Speller, D.C.E., Raghunath, D., Stephens, M., Viant, A.C., Reeves, D.S., Wilkinson, P.J., Broughall, J.M., Holt, H.A. 1976. Epidemic infection by a gentamycin-resistant Staphylococcus aureus in three hospitals. Lancet. 1 : 464.
12. Klastersky, J. 1981. Clinical efficacy of aminoglycosides : an example of balance between microbiology and pharmacology. J. Antimicrob. Chemother. 8 : Suppl. A. 143.

ANTIOBIOTIC RESISTANCE IN VARIOUS MUNICIPALITIES IN THE NETHERLANDS

M.F. MICHEL

To obtain some insight into the magnitude of the resistance problem, several groups of individuals were recently investigated in The Netherlands. The study was conducted by Dr. J.E. Degener of our department in collaboration with Dr. H.A. Valkenburg of the Department of Epidemiology of the Erasmus University in Rotterdam, and concerned the prevalence of resistance to ampicillin, tetracycline, or sulphamethoxazole of E. coli isolated from faecal specimens. The specimens were collected in several groups of the general population and in certain patients admitted to a municipal hospital in the town of Dordrecht and to the University Hospital in Rotterdam.

In the general population a randomized stratified sample of 624 faecal specimens was collected from individuals aged 6 years and older belonging to a community with 60,000 inhabitants. Under stratification is understood equal representation of various age groups within the sample. Because in this community a randomized sample of individuals younger than 6 years could not be obtained, use was made of 46 faecal specimens from children aged 1-6 years and 57 specimens from infants visiting a Welfare Centre in a neighbouring town.

Resistance was assessed by plating suitable dilutions of the faecal material on appropriate media, i.e., either free of antibiotic or containing ampicillin (30 µg/ml), tetracycline (40 µg/ml), or sulphamethoxazole (100 µg/ml). After incubation and counting of colonies, resistance was expressed as the prevalence of resistance or of predominant resistance of the E. coli flora, the term predominantly referring to specimens in which more than 50% of the E. coli bacteria are resistant to an antibiotic.

Table I.

PREVALENCE OF RESISTANT AND PREDOMINANTLY RESISTANT E. COLI IN FAECAL SPECIMENS OF THE AGE-GROUP OF 6 YEARS AND OLDER

Population	No. of specimens	Percentage E. coli resistant to					
		ampicillin		tetra-cycline		sulphame-thoxazole	
		R	PR	R	PR	R	PR
General	577	24	5	42	12	45*	19*
Municipal hospital							
day 1 (surgery)	23	43	4	39	4	48	13
day 10 (medicine)	47	36	17	34	17	49	28
University hospital							
day 1 (surgery)	19	21	5	32	5	37	10
day 10 (medicine)	40	50	38	50	30	35	25

R = resistant, PR = predominantly resistant
*N = 490, Underlined values = significant at P <0.05 level relative to the population at large.

Table II.

PREVALENCE OF RESISTANT AND PREDOMINANTLY RESISTANT E. COLI IN FAECAL SPECIMENS OF THE 1-6 YEAR AGE-GROUP

Population	No. of specimens	Percentage E. coli resistant to					
		ampicillin		tetra-cycline		sulphame-thoxazole	
		R	PR	R	PR	R	PR
General	46	37	7	57	22	57	30
Municipal hospital							
day 10 (medicine)	23	57	30	26	4	52	35
University hospital							
day 1 (surgery)	25	8		20	4	32	12
day 10 (medicine)	48	46	35	44	17	42	25

R = resistant, PR = predominantly resistant
Underlined values = significant at P <0.05 level relative to the general population.

Table III.

PREVALENCE OF RESISTANT AND PREDOMINANTLY RESISTANT E. COLI IN FAECAL SPECIMENS OF THE 0-1 YEAR AGE GROUP

Population	No. of specimens	Percentage E. coli resistant to: ampicillin		tetra-cycline		sulphame-thoxazole	
		R	PR	R	PR	R	PR
General	57	32	18	34	11	52	16
Municipal hospital							
day 10	19	42	11	32	5	47	21
University hospital							
day 10	56	<u>52</u>	<u>39</u>	34	20	41	34

R = resistant, PR = predominantly resistant
Underlined values = significant at P <0.05 level relative to the general population.

Table I shows the prevalence of resistant and predominantly resistant E. coli in faecal specimens originating from different populations of individuals older than 6 years. In the general population resistance to ampicillin, tetracycline, or sulphamethoxazole ranged from 24 to 48%. Except in the group of patients examined on the 10th day after admission in Rotterdam, no significant increase of resistance was observed after hospitalization.

The prevalence of predominantly resistant E. coli in faecal specimens belonging to different populations aged 6 years and older is also shown in Table I. In the general population the prevalence of predominant resistance to ampicillin, tetracycline, and sulphamethoxazole ranged from 5 to 19 per cent. As expected, these percentages are much lower than the corresponding figures for resistance in general. As can be seen from Table I, the prevalence of predominant resistance increased significantly in several groups of patients who had been hospitalized for a period of 10 days.

The findings for children aged 1-6 years and infants, which are presented in Tables II and III, do not differ essentially from those for the older age groups.

The following conclusions may be drawn from this study. The prevalence of resistance to ampicillin, tetracycline, or sulphamethoxazole found for E. coli isolated from faecal specimens of individuals belonging to various age groups in the general population ranged from 24 to 57%. The prevalence of predominantly resistant E. coli in these individuals was much lower, and with one exception ranged between 5 and 22%. A significant increase of predominantly resistant E. coli was found in several groups of patients of different ages who where examined on the 10th day after admission to the municipal or a university hospital.

Young: I thank Dr. Phillips for quoting me correctly. I would like to stress the fact that in the Table, I have pooled the results of Schimpf and collaborators and our own. I think that this is permissible, because we were using a rather similar protocol to study antimicrobial therapy in neutropenic patients. The point is that if one is looking at individuals with a so-called rapidly fatal disease, one can see that the majority of them will do poorly. On the other hand, if you look at the original McCabe and Jackson report it appears that 70% of the patients treated for Gram-negative rod bacteremia with a non-fatal underlying disease, recovered despite inappropriate anti-microbial therapy. The significance of resistance is most evident in individuals with compromised host defenses. If you look at a report from the pre-antimicrobial era, say the one published by Felty and Kiefer in 1924, it appears that the survival of patients with E. coli bacteremia, was about 70% in the absence of antimicrobial therapy. This percentage is virtually identical to what McCabe and Jackson reported for non-fatal underlying disease treated inappropriately. So my conclusion is that the host is of paramount importance if one looks at the relationship between drug resistance and outcome.

I have a question about Dr. Michel's presentation. If I read the slide correctly, day 1 was a prevalence survey of resistance of a surgical ward and day 10 was a prevalence survey of the medical service. I was wondering whether you have any serial data on the same service documenting change in the prevalence of resistance?

Michel: No, we do not have any serial figures. The idea was that we wanted to make sure that the sample from the patient that was admitted to the hospital would not differ from the sample that was drawn from the general population. Although it does not seem very likely, I admit that bias may have been introduced by taking the samples in different departments on day 1 and day 10.

Goldmann: I think both speakers raised the same very fundamental question, one we face all the time: when looking at the prevalence of resistance to an antibiotic, at what point do you say "I have had enough; this specific drug is not going to be my first-choice drug any longer"? We see this currently in paediatrics with the treatment of otitis media. In Boston, 25% of the Haemophilus influenzae strains are now resistant to ampicillin. This is the reason why our first-choice drug is now cefaclor or trimethoprim-sulphamethoxazole. In this particular situation the issue is not so acute and grave as in the neutropenic patient, where we see a rising prevalence of gentamicin resistance. I would like to ask Dr. Phillips, at what point do you say I have had enough; gentamicin is no longer my first drug, from now on I will use amikacin or, as I gathered from your slide, one of the third-generation cephalosporins?

Phillips: If I could just answer the question about when we have had enough. One of the considerations with respect to gentamicin resistance arises when we run out of space to isolate the patients, in other words, when the effort to keep them separate and to stop cross-infection within the hospital becomes excessive. I suspect that there comes a point when our philosophy is that you can use gentamicin and ampicillin with confidence unless you have prior evidence that the patient has an isolate that is associated with septicemia.

Rubin: I just want to emphasize the importance of pharmacokinetics in this type of analysis. Since we are able to deliver only small amounts of an antimicrobial agent to the meninges, it is obvious that our chances of curing meningitis caused by a relatively insensitive organism are low. But if one is dealing with a urinary-tract infection, one can deliver very high concentrations of an antimicrobial agent to the site of the infection. So when the report from a bacteriological laboratory says resistant, you have to interpret that a bit in terms of the site you are going to treat and the level of delivery of the antibiotic to that site. For instance, we have had considerable experience with a three-gram single dose of amoxycillin as therapy for an uncomplicated urinary-tract infection in women. If it is simple cystitis due to an amoxycillin-sensitive organism, we can cure about 98% of the patients. But even if an amoxycillin-resistant organism like Klebsiella is responsible, we are able to cure 65 to 70% of the patients with this single large dose. The reason why is of course that we can deliver 2000 or 3000 micrograms per ml of the antimicrobial agent into the urine. So the point I should like to add to your comment is that when treatment is initiated, resistance does not tell us the complete story: the pharmacokinetics and the site of infection should be taken into consideration as well.

Phat: On one of your slides, Dr. Phillips, I noticed that probenecid was administered simultaneously with an antimicrobial agent. There is at least one publication indicating that probenecid hinders not only excretion of a drug but also its transfer to the tissues. Shouldn't this be interpreted as an example of pharmacokinetic hindrance?

Phillips: One should realize that if probenicid hinders the transfer of the drug to the tissues somewhat, it also has a raising effect on the level of the drug in the blood. Therefore, when probenecid is used it is difficult to predict what the level of the drug at the site of the infection will be.

ANTIBIOTIC PRESCRIBING IN A GENERAL HOSPITAL

FIONA MOSS

Antibiotics are used throughout general hospitals and are prescribed to about one third of patients admitted to hospital. The emergence of antibiotic resistant bacteria has drawn attention to the quality of antibiotic prescribing in hospital practice. Wanton use of antimicrobial therapy unnecessarily increases the risk of the development of antibiotic resistant bacteria.

One way to find out if antibiotics are being over-used or misused is to carry out a survey of antibiotic prescribing or antibiotic audit. If antibiotic misuse is identified then it is only understanding why the prescribers have prescribed these antimicrobial agents that any attempt to improve antibiotic prescribing habits can be made.

The Central Middlesex Hospital is a 480 bedded district general hospital in North West London. There are acute medical and surgical services as well as regional opthalmic and regional neurosurgical units. It was decided to carry out a survey of antibiotic prescribing at this Hospital for a four week period during November 1978. The aims of the survey were threefold. Firstly to establish the patterns of antibiotic prescribing, secondly to find out the reasons for antibiotic use and thirdly to make some assessment of the quality of antibiotic prescribing.

THE SURVEY

Previous surveys have determined the reasons for antibiotic use from data in patients' notes. Not only is this an indirect method of finding out why clinicians prescribe antibiotics, but it is a notoriously incomplete and possibly inaccurate source of information. The prescriber, however, should be able to give a first hand and accurate account of the reasons for antibiotic use. This survey was therefore based on an interview with the prescriber of each prescription. This provided direct information about the reasons for prescribing antibiotics and was used as the basis for qualitative assessment of prescribing habits.

THE INTERVIEWS

The first step in obtaining the prescriber orientated data was to record prescriptions of antibiotics as they were written. Every new prescription of an antibiotic was noted and details of the patient were taken from records. As soon as possible after this the prescriber was interviewed. The aim of the interview was to find out the reason for the prescription and also to get some insight into the thinking which had prompted the prescription. A standard questionnaire was used. The prescribers were first asked to state whether the prescription of the antibiotic was therapeutic or prophylactic in intent. Prescribers of therapeutic prescriptions were then asked to state the site of infection, the evidence for infection at that site, whether the bacteria responsible for the infection had been isolated and, if not, to state the suspected infecting agent, and whether there were any other features relevant to the diagnosis of infection (e.g. diabetes, in-dwelling catheters). A different questionnaire was used to assess antibiotic prophylaxis. The prescribers of prophylactic prescriptions were asked to state whether the patient was exposed to any special risk of infection such as operative procedure and to give its nature and date, whether the patient had any condition which might enhance susceptibility to infection (e.g. immunological deficiency, broken mechanical barriers such as CSF leak, rheumatic heart disease) and to state the potential infecting agents against which the prophylaxis was directed.

EXTENT OF ANTIBIOTIC PRESCRIBING

Antibiotics were prescribed to 28 % of patients admitted to the hospital. A similar proportion of medical surgical patients received these drugs.

TYPES OF ANTIBIOTICS PRESCRIBED

The type of antibiotics used differed from previously reported surveys. The penicillins accounted for over 60 % of the antibiotics prescribed, with Ampicillin being the most frequently used single drug (Table 1). No other survey has found a high proportion of Ampicillin use. This contrasts with the use of cephalosporins, which accounted for less than 5 % of the antibiotics prescribed.

Table 1.
SITES OF INFECTION FOR WHICH ANTIBIOTICS WERE PRESCRIBED BY MAJOR SPECIALITIES

SITE	MEDICINE	SURGERY	OBSTETRICS	TOTAL
Lower respiratory tract (chest)	86	22	0	108
Urinary tract	22	28	6	56
Genital tract	2	14	9	25
Wound	0	19	0	19*
Abdominal-gastro-intestinal tract	5	10	0	15
Skin and subcutaneous tissue	7	8	0	15
Upper respiratory tract	8	3	0	11
Other	20	10	0	30
TOTAL	150	114	15	279

*Includes 17 surgical wounds

REASONS FOR ANTIBIOTIC PRESCRIBING

The prescribers stated that over 70 % of the antibiotic courses were prescribed for the treatment of infection and the rest was for prophylaxis. The surgical services were responsible for almost all the courses of antibiotic prophylaxis.

THERAPEUTIC ANTIBIOTIC USE

Lower respiratory tract infection and urinary tract infection were the two most frequent sites of infection for which antibiotics were prescribed, together accounting for almost 60 % of the sites of infection, identified by the prescribers (Table 2).

Table 2.
TYPES OF ANTIBIOTICS

ANTIBIOTIC	NUMBER OF PRESCRIPTIONS
Ampicillin*	213 (41 %)
Cloxacillin**	57 (11 %)
Penicillin	48 (9 %)
Co-trimoxazole	47 (9 %)
Metronidazole	37 (7 %)
Chloramphenicol	26 (5 %)
Cephaloridine***	19 (4 %)
Gentamicin	19 (4 %)
Erythromycin	14 (3 %)

Other antibiotics used were : nystatin 9, cefuroxime 7, amphotericin 6, neomycin 6, sulphadimidine 4, sodium fusidate 3, oxytetracycline 3, nitrofurantoin 3, doxycycline 1, nalidixic acid 1, tobramycin 1.
*Includes amoxycillin,
**includes flucloxacillin,
***includes cephradine.

PROPHYLACTIC ANTIBIOTIC USE

Less than half of these prescriptions were for "convential surgical prophylaxis", that is, for prevention of systemic or local infection at the time of operation. Other reasons for "prophylaxis" included prescription for antibiotics as a response to peri-operative events or findings, trauma, including prescription following compound fractures and skull fractures complicated by CSF leak.

ASSESSMENT OF ANTIBIOTIC PRESCRIBING

Therapeutic antibiotic use

Assessment of therapeutic antibiotic prescribing was done in two ways ; first the appropriateness of the choice of the antibiotics for the site of infection was assessed and secondly the need for antibiotic use was assessed on the basis of the evidence of infection.

Antibiotic choice was assessed by a consultant physician and a consultant microbiologist. They considered that 80 % of antibiotics were appropiate treatment for infection at the stated site. Although this may seem to be quite a good result for the prescribers, some of the inappropriate choices were potentially dangerous. In particular, some prescriptions provided inadequate cover for likely infecting agents.

It was only possible to make an assessment of the need for anti biotic use for infection at two sites: lower respiratory tract infections and urinary tract infections. These infections accounted for 60 % of the infections treated with antibiotics. The diagnosis of infection at these sites depends on different types of information and clinical decision taking. Lower respiratory tract infection is diagnosed on clinical evidence whereas the diagnosis of urinary tract infection can be confirmed or refuted by objective microbiological tests. The interviews with the prescribers, relevant chest X rays and laboratory data were used for the qualitative assessment of antibiotic need.

Lower respiratory tract infection (LRTI)

Over 8 % of patients admitted to hospital were treated for LRTI. This description included patients who had pneumonia as well as those who had infective exacerbation of chronic bronchitis. A system of scoring both respiratory and non-respiratory features of infection was devised (Table 3). This included features important to the diagnosis of both pneumonia and bronchitis. Most of the information was obtained from the survey data but it was extended to include chest X ray data and leucocyte counts collected after the survey, but which were available to the prescriber at the time of prescription. The chest X rays were reported and scored independently from the survey data by a consultant chest physician. The total score from all these features was used as an "Index of Infection" for 94 adult patients, who were prescribed anti-biotics for the treatment of chest infection.

Table 3.

METHOD USED TO SCORE FEATURES INDICATIVE OF LOWER RESPIRATORY TRACT INFECTION. TOTAL SCORE = "INDEX OF INFECTION"

	SCORE		
FEATURE	0	1	2
RESPIRATORY			
Sputum*	Mucoid	-	Purulent
Function**	No change	Deteriorating	-
X rays***	No evidence of infection	Abnormalities possibly due to infection	Abnormalities unequivocally suggestive of infection
NON-RESPIRATORY			
Temperatures †	$< 37^{o}$ C	37° C-38.5^{o} C	$> 38.5^{o}$ C
Leucocyte count ∇	$< 11X10^{9}/1$	$11-16X10^{9}/1$	$> 16X10^{9}/1$
General state**	-	Ill	Very ill/toxic
Diabetes †	Not present	Well controlled	Worsening control of ketoacidosis
Steroid therapy †	-	Long term	-

*Where prescribers and laboratory assessment differed - the higher score was used.
**Based on prescriber's statement.
***Chest X rays taken on the day of prescription or within the preceding 24 h were reviewed without clinical information.
† Taken from the original survey data.
∇ Taken directly from laboratory copies of haematology reports.

The possible range of the "Index of Infection" was from 0 to 14. Antibiotic use was considered justified for patients whose index of infection was 3 or more and included at least one point from a respiratory feature. If the index was 2 and included a respiratory feature the use of antibiotics was considered questionable. Other prescriptions were considered unjustified.

Less than half the antibiotics prescribed for lower respiratory tract infections were considered justified. The actual scores ranged from 0 to 8 (Table 4). Justified antibiotic use included patients expectorating purulent sputum who were short of breath as well as the patient whose index of infection was 8, who had high fever, was collapsed, had a moderately raised leucocyte count, was short of breath and whose chest X ray showed consolidation.

Table 4.
INDICES OF INFECTION FOR 94 ADULT PATIENTS

INDEX OF INFECTION									
0	1	2	3	4	5	6	7	8	Total
15	18	15	10	16	12	4	3	1	94

Forty percent of antibiotics prescribed for lower respiratory tract infection were considered unjustified. These included 15 patients whose index of infection was 0. In clinical terms this means that these patients were apyrexial, did not have raised leucocyte counts, were not expectorating purulent sputum, were not described by the prescribers as having deteriorating respiratory function and did not have chest X rays suggestive of infection.

The "Index of Infection" identified a problem, namely that antibiotics were prescribed unnecessarily for respiratory tract infection as a result of inadequate assessment of the evidence of infection. The data from the interviews with the prescribers provided the reasons for inappropriate prescriptions. Each prescriber had been asked to state his evidence of infection. For nine patients with an "Index of Infection" of 0 the prescriber stated that his evidence of infection was chest X ray changes. These chest X rays were reported by the independent assessor - none was found to have changes, judged by the assessor, to be infective in origin. Most of them showed changes of pulmonary oedema. Similar misinterpretation of chest X ray changes was found in patients with scores of 1. In other patients with an "Index of Infection" of 0 the evidence for respiratory tract infection was that they were simply in congestive cardiac failure. Other patients were prescribed antibiotics on the basis of expectoration of mucoid sputum and abnormal lung sounds. One prescriber even admitted to being uncertain about the reasons for the diagnosis.

A significantly higher proportion of the antibiotics prescribed for LRTI to patients over 71 years than to younger patients were considered unjustified. Signs of infection may be more subtle in the elderly, but even this cannot justify the misuse of antibiotics demonstrated at the Central Middlesex Hospital. One of the patients prescribed antibiotics for respiratory tract infection had been admitted with acute left ventricular failure ; the notes revealed that she had been admitted on several previous occasions with similar signs and symptoms and had been treated successfully with diuretics but without antibiotics by other doctors. The use of antibiotics in addition to diuretics on this occasion was undeniably unnecessary.

Urinary tract infection (UTI)

Urine specimens from all patients with UTI had been sent to the laboratory for bacteriological examination and copies of the reports sent to clinicians were available. Prescribers' statements about the clinical evidence of infections was available from the interview data. The clinical and bacteriological data were used together to assess the need for antibiotic use for 55 patients who had been prescribed antibiotics for treatment of UTI.

Almost half those treated for UTI, 26 patients, were prescribed antibiotics without bacteriological evidence of infection. Of these 7,patients were prescribed antibiotics although reports stating that urine was sterile were available to the prescriber at the time of diagnosis. For a further 11 patients reports were subsequently available which stated that the urine was sterile.

Although the prescribers sent urine specimens for bacteriological examination from all patients with UTI their inability to act on negative results suggests a ritualistic approach to laboratory investigation which invalidates their using these tests.

The rest of the patients were prescribed antibiotics following isolation of bacteria from urine. Nine of these patients, four of whom had urinary catheters in situ, had no clinical symptoms of UTI nor of generalised infection, but were prescribed antibiotics in response to the isolation of bacteria from a single routine urine specimen.

Thus for 27 patients, almost half of those treated, it was considered that either initiation or continuation of antibiotic therapy was unjustified.

Prophylactic antibiotic use

Assessment of antibiotic prophylaxis was limited to the 55 prescriptions of "conventional surgical prophylaxis". As there is no clear consensus about the indications for antibiotic surgical prophylaxis the assessment of prophylaxis was confined to the following features : (a) time of prophylaxis, which should be just before the start of the procedure (b) the drug used, which should be adequate to cover for the likely infecting agents for the stated procedure (c) the route of administration, which should be parenteral except for Metronidazole, which is effective as a rectal preparation and (d) the planned duration, which should be no longer than 24 hours.

Only 7 % of prescriptions were judged as correct for all 4 criteria. The commonest error was the excessive intended duration of antibiotic prophylaxis with 80 % of these prescriptions being intended to be continued for more than 24 hours. In contrast to the choice of antibiotic for therapeutic use the choice of antibiotic for prophylaxis was considered correct for only 45 % of prescriptions.

Analysis of the quality of antibiotic prescribing

An unacceptably high proportion of antibiotics used at the Central Middlesex Hospital were prescribed unnecessarily. Almost half the antibiotics prescribed for LRTI and UTI were considered unjustified. Inadequate clinical assessment and poor use of laboratory investigations were the main features contributing to unnecessary therapeutic use of antibiotics. The use of antibiotics for prophylaxis was unsatisfactory with extensive duration being the most frequent prescribing error.

The apparent good choice of antibiotic seems to have been based on knowing which antibiotics are "good for the site" rather than any understanding of the organism likely to be the cause of the infection. Less than 20 % of therapeutic antibiotics were prescribed as the result of the isolation of bacteria. For half of the remaining antibiotic courses the prescribers were unable to state a likely infecting agent for the infection they were treating. Whilst ignorance may not matter in most instances, two patients included in the survey became seriously ill because antibiotics prescribed were inadequate cover for the infection being treated. Rational antibiotic prescribing cannot be expected if the prescribers have no concept of a likely infecting agent.

There is in operation at the Central Middlesex Hospital a "non-prescriptive antibiotic policy". The reports of antibiotic sensitivities of bacteria isolated from culture of specimens sent to the laboratory which are issued to the clinicians are limited to certain antibiotics. Sensitivity of bacteria to cephalosporins is not reported to the prescriber unless the organism is resistant to the hospital's "first line" antibiotic. No direct influence is exerted on the prescribers' antibiotic choice, but the range of antibiotics actually prescribed in the hospital suggests that indirect methods are very effective in controlling the types of antibiotics used in a hospital.

It is interesting to note that the use of Cefuroxime, then a recent addition to the antimicrobial pharmacy, was related to the presence in the Hospital of a pharmaceutical firm representative. In the light of their poor use of antibiotics and their lack of understanding about likely infecting agents, the prescribers' capability of understanding information issued from pharmaceutical companies mus be questioned.

The prescriptions were all written by junior hospital doctors whose lack of experience may have been the cause of the unnecessary prescriptions, prescribing antibiotics on a "just in case" basis without making an accurate clinical assessment. Only one prescription was subsequently stopped by a consultant so reinforcing behaviour patterns and lack of thought preceding the decision to prescribe an antibiotic. The apparent reluctance of the consultant staff to stop unnecessary prescriptions of antibiotics suggests that either they endorse decisions about evidence of infection made by their juniors or they do not participate in the decision to prescribe antibiotics, or that the tradition of an antibiotic course being continued once it has been started adds to the psychological difficulty of scoring out someone else's prescription. Awareness by the consultant staff of the extent of unnecessary antibiotic prescribing throughout the hospital might reduce the prescriptions of antibiotics made by their juniors.

The unwanted effects of the poor clinical decision taking which results in unjustified antibiotic use are not confined to the covert danger of the unnecessary increase in the risk of the emergence of antibiotic resistant bacteria. As was seen in one patient included in this survey the label of a diagnosis of infection, when not appropriate, may have serious adverse effects. In spite of evidence to the contrary, this patient was diagnosed as having a urinary tract infection and was prescribed antibiotics. This resulted in an almost fatal delay in recognising serious abdominal pathology.

The solution to the problem of antibiotic prescribing which have been encountered in this survey lie in improved medical education at both undergraduate and postgraduate levels. The task belongs as much to the clinicians as to the microbiologists and pharmacologists. The teaching of bacteriology must be combined with clinical teaching ; the patient with a lobar pneumonia rather than an agar plate should be the point of reference for the teaching about Streptococcus pneumoniae. The separation of the laboratory from the arena of clinical decision making is illustrated by the wealth of information about antibiotic prescribing which is available but hidden from clinicians as it is mostly published in bacteriological journals. Antibiotic policies are unlikely to have any further influence on antibiotic prescribing than that which we have seen as an unobtrusive policy at present in operation at the Central Middlesex Hospital.

INSIGHTS INTO ANTIBACTERIAL PHARMACOTHERAPY AND MEASURES LEADING TO CONTROL OF DRUG USE

C.W.R. PHAF

Measures to control antibacterial pharmacotherapy (1-3) developed by clinical microbiologists and work done by clinical pharmacists are complementary. One function of clinical pharmacy -- or patient-oriented pharmacy -- is to provide the means for appropriate pharmacotherapy, i.e., the drugs and the information and organization necessary to use them properly. I once heard a simple definition of this field: clinical pharmacy is finding out where the stuff goes. That is exactly what we try to do with respect to antibacterial pharmacotherapy.

Since the restrictions of a short paper do not permit a detailed discussion of our methods and results, I shall attempt only to give an impression of the approaches we use to gain insight into patterns of drug use. Further information can be found in the relevant literature (4-8).

The total consumption of antibacterial medication can be expressed as cost price, corrected for inflation, per patient-day and as a percentage of the total drug costs (9) (Fig. 1).If "nature" is allowed to take its course, 40 to 50% of the total drug costs in a general hospital will be accounted for by antibacterial drugs. With a great deal of effort, it may be possible to reduce this figure to about 20% or even less.

The use of specific groups of antibacterials can be expressed as cost price; the percentage of the total cost price taken by antibacterial pharmacotherapy can be expressed as units of use and as a percentage of total units of use (10)(Fig. 2).
The frequency of prescription of specific preparations or the number of orders for antibacterial pharmotherapy can be shown in cumulative plots (4,5). The latter method indicates who the users

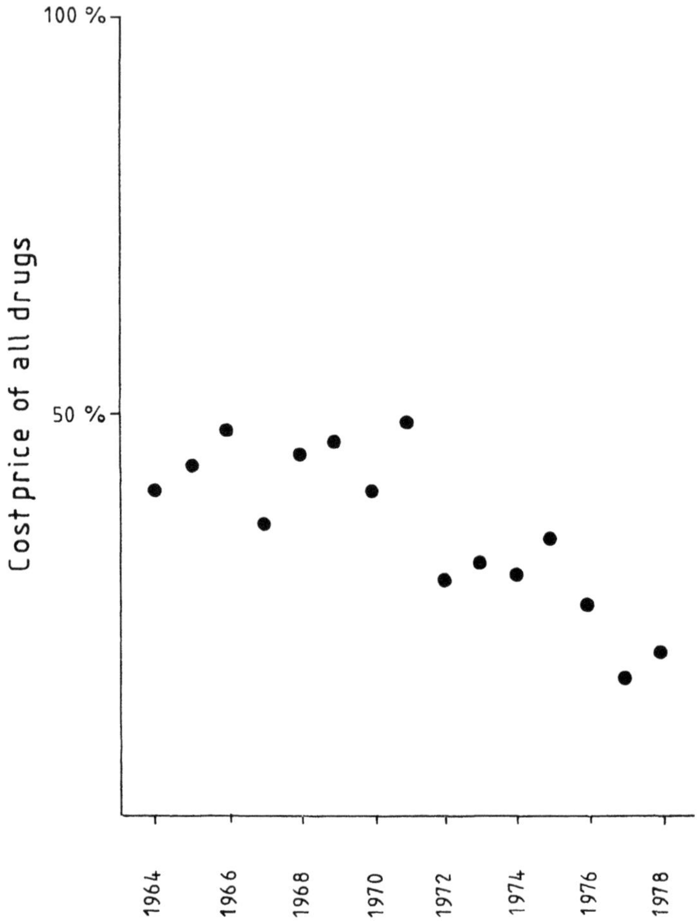

Fig. 1. Per cent cost price of antibacterial drugs.

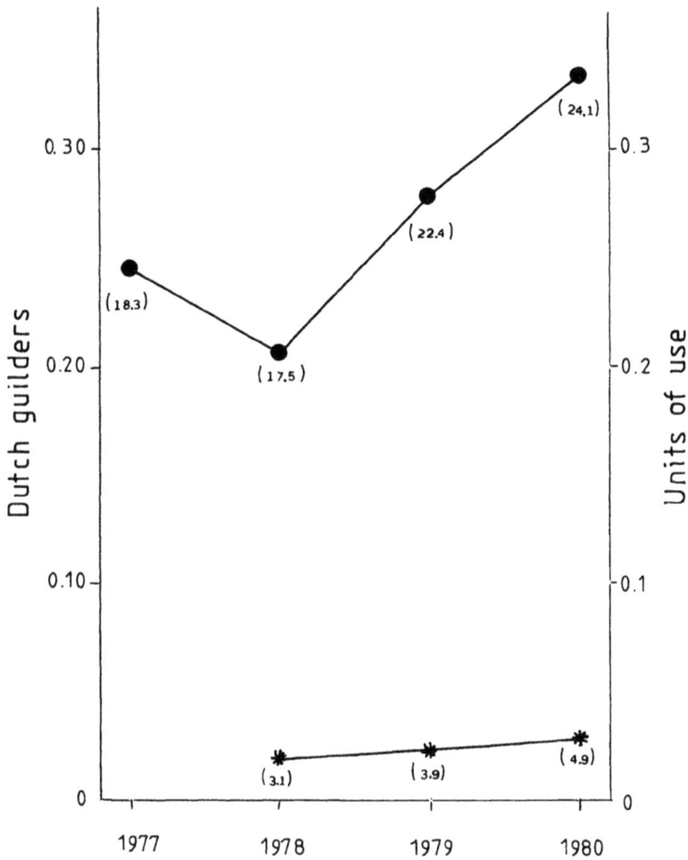

Fig. 2. Costs of aminoglycosides (●) and units (★) used per patient day. Values in parentheses give for aminoglycosides the percentage of total antibiotic costs or total units of antimicrobial drugs used.

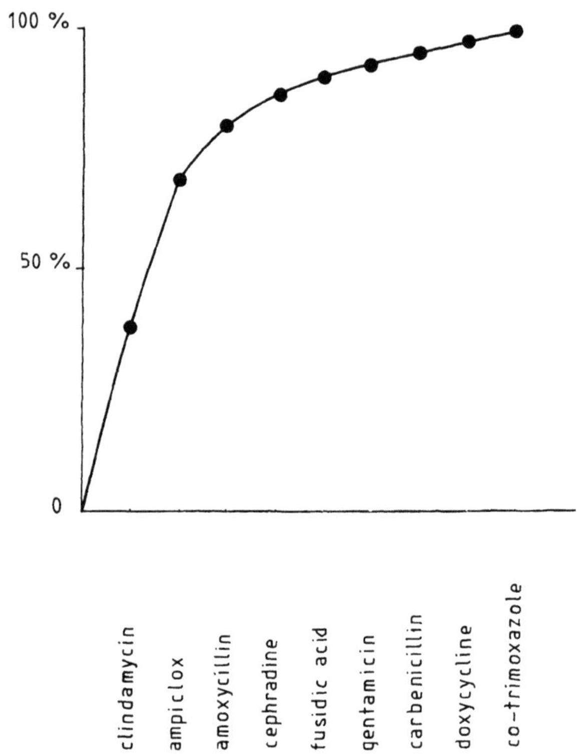

Fig. 3. Prescribing of antimicrobial drugs by the Department of Orthopaedics (cumulative percentages).

of a specific preparation are (i.e., the departments of otorhinolaryngology, ophthalmology, and dermatology) and which preparations are used by whom (Fig. 3).

The next question is: how are specific preparations used, for what indications, and on the basis of what data? Are, for instance, gentamicin and tobramycin properly used (9,10) (Table I)? How are specific infections treated (Table II)? What is done with our advice; sometimes it has effect (Table III), sometimes not (Table IV).

Table I.

TREATMENT WITH GENTAMICIN AND TOBRAMYCIN

	1978	1979	1980
Total number of patients in two months	26	19	23
after culture result	13	7	5
while awaiting culture result	4	5	7
contradictory to culture result	9	7	10

Table II.

TREATMENT OF PSEUDOMONAS INFECTIONS

	1978	1979	1980
Total number of infections in two months	33	12	21
superinfections	27	5	6
treatment adequate	12	5	6
treatment not adequate	21	7	15

Table III.

MOST FREQUENTLY USED ANTIBACTERIALS - DEPARTMENT OF SURGERY

	Number of patients treated		
	1978	1979	1980
penicillin and streptomycin	7		
ampiclox*	9		
amoxycillin	19	8	13
gentamicin and tobramycin		10	

* ampicillin plus cloxacillin

Table IV.

MOST FREQUENTLY USED ANTIBACTERIALS - DEPARTMENT OF UROLOGY

	Number of patients treated		
	1978	1979	1980
penicillin and streptomycin	29	9	10
amoxycillin	24	7	21
co-trimoxazole	10	2	11
hydroxymethylnitrofurantoïn	7	10	13
nalidixic acid	20		

It seems clear that restrictive measures are necessary. In this respect, a formulary regimen has proven to be very useful (8). Non-formulary drugs are not dispensed unless the physician who signs for the request provides arguments satisfactory to the relevant ad hoc committee.

In daily practice, the hospital pharmacists check and guide the requests. We do this by the use of special forms. Such forms enable us to register arguments and answers to requests, provide an accessible record of answers, and facilitate analysis of changes in use patterns. In 1980, 24% of the exceptional requests for antibacterial preparations were refused; in 1981, this figure was 17%; and in the first three month of 1982 it was 12.5%.

The system itself has of course a limiting effect. More people think twice before they prescribe when they know they are being watched. The medical world would be better and more comfortable if consultation and natural teamwork led to optimal quality, but daily practice shows that this is not enough (5,7). It is not sufficient to remind people of the fact that specialistic advice must never be ignored. We need compulsory rules; we need medical auditing.

REFERENCES

1. Moss, F., McSwiggan, D.A., McNicol, M.W., Miller, D.L. 1981. Survey of antibiotic prescribing in a district general hospital. I: Pattern of use. Lancet ii: 349.
2. Moss, F., McSwiggan, D.A., McNicol, M.W., Miller, D.L. 1981. Survey of antibiotic prescribing in a district general hospital. II: Lower respiratory tract infection. Lancet ii: 407.

3. Moss, F., McSwiggan, D.A., McNicol, M.W., Miller, D.L. 1981. Survey of antibiotic prescribing in a district general hospital. III: Urinary tract infection. Lancet ii: 461.
4. Phaf, C.W.R. 1977. On policy of antibiotic use control. Medisch Magazine TGO/JDR 2: 41/15, 48/22.
5. Phaf, C.W.R. 1977. Clinical pharmaceutical audit and antibacterial pharmaceutical audit of antibacterial pharmacotherapy. In: Clinical Pharmacy. Eds E. van der Kleijn, J.R. Jonkers. Elsevier/North Holland Biomedical Press. Amsterdam. 179.
6. Phaf, C.W.R. 1978. A policy for the control of antibiotic use. J. Clin. Pharm. 3: 119.
7. Phaf, C.W.R. 1979. Retrospective and prospective drug use review of antibacterial pharmacotherapy. In: Progress in Clinical Pharmacy. Eds I.D. Schaaf, E. van der Kleijn. Elsevier/North Holland Biomedical Press. Amsterdam. 207.
8. Phaf, C.W.R. 1980. The role of clinical pharmacy in medical audit. J. Clin. Hosp. Pharm. 5: 269.
9. Phaf, C.W.R. 1980. Development of the role of clinical pharmacy in medical audit. In: Progress in Clinical Pharmacy. II. Eds G. Aulagner, J.C. Plasse, E. van der Kleijn. Elsevier/North Holland Biomedical Press. Amsterdam. 17.
10. Phaf, C.W.R. 1982. The impact of formulary and pharmacotherapy committee policy on use-patterns of drugs. In: Proceedings Workshop on Clinical Pharmacy, Catwick, March 11-13, 1981. In press.

DISCUSSION EDITED BY C.W.R. PHAF

Mattie: The fact that prescribers have the feeling of being watched often has a limiting effect on prescribing habits. Was any influence or trend observable in the results during the survey that might have been caused by the course of the trial itself?

Moss: People knew about the survey in advance. Nevertheless, there was no trend. During the 28 days of the survey, the bad prescriptions of antibiotics were the same at the end as they were at the beginning. I did not comment on the prescriptions during the survey, and I do not believe that I changed antibiotic prescribing habits during the survey. If I had influenced the prescribing of antibiotics, I presume that I would have made physicians prescribe less. We did a pilot trial lasting a week before starting the survey and found no difference in the amount of antibiotics prescribed during the week without an interview and the weeks of the interviews.

Hudson: The solution to the problem is: good and appropriate medical education. Formal quality-assurance programs can also effectuate improvement of prescribing patterns.

Moss: Many patients don't really need the antibiotics that are prescribed. This represents an unnecessary risk of resistance and unnecessarily high costs. Prescribers would be more aware of such covered "side effects" if the patients developed a rash.

van den Broek: Did you observe any difference in prescribing habits after the results of your study were published?

Moss: We did not repeat the study, so we could not get such information.

Goldmann: We introduced a special form on which physicians had to indicate whether antibiotics were prescribed prophylactically, empirically for a pathogen yet to be identified, or for therapeutic purposes. We stopped antibiotics after 48 hours for the prophylactic, 72 hours for the empiric, and 7 days for the therapeutic administration. Physicians had to rewrite the order if they wanted to continue. This method caused a dramatic decline in the duration of antibiotic prophylaxis and there was also a decline in the percentage of patients receiving prophylaxis. Such regulative measures were effective. Education alone may not be sufficient.

van Furth: In Leiden we have a restrictive antibiotic policy and a uniform agreement on prophylactic use. At the moment, we are trying to get the written agreement of all the physicians for regimens for specific kinds of infections.

Jackson: We have made good progress as to the reduction of the duration of antibiotic prophylaxis in surgery. Intra-operative prophylaxis is perhaps all that is necessary. We found that 80% of the patients who had suffered a previous hypersensitivity reaction to beta-lactam antibiotics, had not been asked whether they had had a reaction before the drug was prescribed.

Moss: At the interview, prescribers were certainly not always aware of antibiotic sensitivities to be expected.

ANTIMICROBIAL RESISTANCE IN HOSPITAL: NEW TRENDS AND CONTROL

R.A. WEINSTEIN

INTRODUCTION

Since the 1960's reports of antibiotic resistance in hospitals have appeared with increasing frequency. Prior to 1965 no hospital epidemics involving multiply resistant gram-negative bacilli were investigated by the United States' Center for Disease Control. However, during 1965-1975 11 of the 15 nosocomial outbreaks of Enterobacteriaceae that were studied involved multiply resistant strains (1). Among gram-positive bacteria, resistance of Staphylococcus aureus to penicillin became epidemic in the early 1960's and ultimately has come to be considered the norm. Since the late 1960's outbreaks of methicillin resistant S. aureus have been reported, first from Europe and more recently from the United States. Nosocomial resistance has become so commonplace that it is often overlooked until it is either extreme or epidemic. In this paper, we present interventions that may help hospitals avoid such catastrophies.

DEFINITION OF MULTIPLE RESISTANCE ; MECHANISMS AND GENETICS

Definition

Multiple resistance in bacteria may be arbitrarily defined as resistance to two or more unrelated antibiotics to which the bacteria are usually susceptible. Alternatively, resistance to certain key or first-line drugs may be used as a marker for problems with drug resistance, e.g., methicillin resistance in S. aureus or aminoglycoside (gentamicin, tobramycin, or amikacin) resistance in gram-negative bacilli.

Mechanisms

The most common mechanisms of resistance include production by bacteria of antibiotic inactivating enzymes, such as penicillinases or aminoglycoside modifying enzymes ; changes in cell wall permeability or uptake of antibiotics ; alteration in target sites, such as ribosomes ; changes in susceptible metabolic pathways ; or changes in cell wall binding sites that prevent antibiotic attachment (2).

Genetics

Chromosomal versus plasmid resistance. Resistance may be mediated either by the bacterial chromosome or by extra-chromosomal DNA (2). Chromosomal resistance occurs by spontaneous mutation and Darwinian selection of organisms resistant to single (or closely related) agents. In contrast, bacteria may acquire resistance by the acrual of extra-chromosomal DNA (plasmids) called R factors or resistance plasmids, which often encode multiple resistances to unrelated drugs. Plasmids may spread rapidly across species lines and even between genera. An example of the extensive spread of resistance plasmids is the presence of the same plasmid-mediated TEM-1 beta-lactamase - an enzyme that confers resistance to ampicillin - in a variety of gram-negative bacteria, including Enterobacteriaceae, gonococci and Hemophilus influenza.

Transposons. At the molecular level, portions of plasmids, called transposons, may hitch-hike from one plasmid to another or between plasmid and bacterial chromosome. Transposons carrying genes for resistance may align with other elements, such as those encoding virulence or colonization factors, creating plasmids with an awesome one-two punch.

ENDEMIC SPREAD OF RESISTANT BACTERIA IN HOSPITALS

Significant factors which lead to the endemic occurrence of multiple drug resistant bacteria in hospitals are shown schematically in Figure 1 and are described below in order of approximate importance.

Hands of personnel

In the hospital, bacteria may spread indirectly from person-to-person by transient carriage on hands of hospital personnel. Such spread may result in large numbers of colonized patients whose normal pharyngeal or intestinal flora is replaced by multiply resistant enteric bacilli or Pseudomonas. Extensive spread of resistant strains (the submerged portion of the iceberg) may occur before clinical problems (the tip of the iceberg) are recognized.

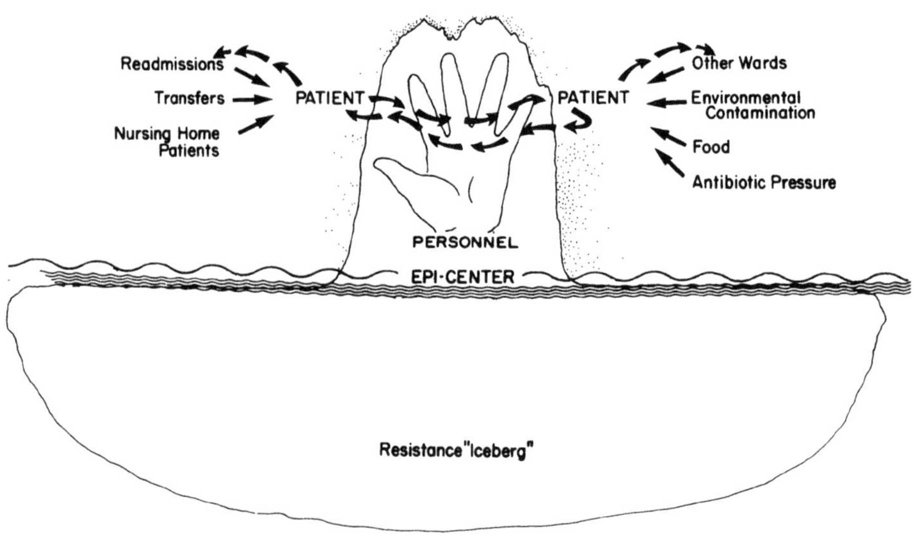

Figure 1. The dynamics of nosocomial resistance (see text). (Reproduced with persmission from Weinstein et al. (16)).

Admissions

Admission (or readmission) of patients with preexisting gastrointestinal, genitourinary, respiratory, or wound colonization (or infection) with resistant strains has accounted for up to 25 % of the aminoglycoside resistant gram-negative bacilli in our hospital (3). Such carriage may result from prior hospitalization or from residence in institutions such as nursing homes. Urinary tract infections with multiply resistant Proteus and Providencia appear to be a particular problem among nursing home patients admitted with chronic indwelling catheters.

Antibiotics

Antibiotic pressures may suppress sensitive flora and facilitate colonization of patients by more resistant bacteria. Because of R factors, use of one antibiotic may allow resistance to several unrelated agents to co-emerge. Antibiotics may also select a resistant subpopulation of bacteria from a larger sensitive population. In a recent scenario we have seen use of the "second generation" cephalosporin, cephamandole, for treatment of sensitive Enterobacter infections select out strains resistant to both cephamandole and "third generation" drugs.

Environment

Resistant organisms may spread via environmental contamination, especially of patient care equipment like urine measuring devices. Serratia has appeared particularly adept at this type of spread, causing extensive asymptomic urinary tract infections (and possible perineal and/or intestinal colonization) before significant clinical problems are noted.

Other sources

The source of approximately 20 % of resistant gram-negative bacilli is unknown. Factors of possible but generally unproven importance include : 1) foodborne contamination ; 2) airborne contamination, which is rarely related to gram-negative bacilli ; 3) contamination of the inanimate environment, such as sink drains, with which patients do not come directly into contact ; and 4) personnel disseminators of resistant bacteria. Although transient hand carriage of nosocomial gram-negative bacilli by personnel is common, persistent carriage and dissemination is rare. Such dissemination by personnel is much more likely to occur with gram-positive cocci, which may colonize nasal mucosa ; perineal, rectal, or axillary folds ; and other sites.

EPIDEMIC SPREAD OF MULTIPLY RESISTANT BACTERIA IN HOSPITALS

Characteristics

Outbreaks of multiple drug resistant bacteria are usually due to indirect person-to-person spread of infection on the hands of hospital personnel (4). Less often, common-source outbreaks or epidemics due to personnel disseminators, particularly of Staphylococci, occur. Table 1 lists the characteristics of several person-to person outbreaks of multiply resistant urinary tract infections.

Precipitating events

The events leading to any nosocomial epidemic are probably multifactorial. In most outbreaks of multiple drug resistant bacteria, precipitating factors have not been well elucidated. Factors that could increase person-to-person spread include poor aseptic practices, as in crowded units or when the nurse-to-patient ratio becomes too low. Spread from the environment is facilitated by poor housekeeping practices that lead to reservoirs of resistant organisms within the hospital, as when infected urine is allowed to remain in urine measuring or testing devices. Excessive use of antibiotics may increase the selective pressure for resistant strains. Certain fortuitous events may precipitate outbreaks, such as contamination of a commercial product, admission of a patient who is a heavy shedder of multiply resistant bacteria, or acquisition of resistance by a bacterial species that is adept at colonization or unusually resistant to disinfection. Also, advances in medical care, like transplantation, dialysis and new prosthetic devices, always create additional epidemic risks.

Table 1. EPIDEMIOLOGIC PATTERNS IN OUTBREAKS OF URINARY TRACT INFECTION BY MULTIPLY RESISTANT ORGANISMS

Factor	Organisms*		
	Klebsiella pneumoniae	Serratia marcescens	Proteus rettgeri
Reservoir			
Symptomatic GU[†] infection	++++	±	++
Asymptomatic GU infection	++	++++	+++
Gastrointestinal colonization	++	0	0
Mode of transmission	Hands[§]	Hands	Hands
Spatial clustering of cases prominent	++	++++	++++
Risk factors			
Urinary catheterization	Yes	Yes	Yes
Broad-spectrum antimicrobial exposure	Yes	Yes	Yes
Urinary catheter irrigation	Yes	No	No
GU instrumentation	No	No	Yes

*Scale: 0 (no contribution) to ++++ (maximal contribution).
†GU = genitourinary.
§Indirect contact spread on hands of personnel.

(Adapted from Schaberg, Weinstein, & Stamm (4)).

Epi-centers

Certain areas within the hospital, especially intensive care units (ICUs) and burn, neurosurgical and urology units, are prone to outbreaks. These areas house acutely ill patients who are subjected to many invasive procedures and often exposed to multiple antibiotics under circumstances in which asepsis may occasionally be trampled in the rush of crisis care. We have found that such units represent "epi-centers" (fig. 1) in which multiply resistant bacteria may breed. As colonized patients are transferred throughout the hospital from such epi-centers, they may leave a trail of resistance.

PLASMID (AND TRANSPOSON) OUTBREAKS

Examples

Most outbreaks that have been described have been due to epidemic spread of single strains. However, in the past five years several "plasmid outbreaks" have been described in which a resistance plasmid has caused either simultaneous or sequential resistance to occur in epidemic fashion in different species or genera (Table 2) (5-8). We are also recognizing that transposition of plasmid segments (or other spatial rearrangements of genetic material) may lead to "transposon outbreaks" involving whole families of related resistance plasmids (9).

Table 2. EXAMPLES OF PLASMID OUTBREAKS*

Setting	Bacteria (no.)	Predominant Infections	Appearance of Resistance (duration)	Plasmid-borne Resistances
Neonatal ICU (5)	Klebsiella Serotype 30 (19) Serotype 19 (6)	NS	Sequential (9 mo; 5 mo)	Gm,kn,am,cf,cb
Hospital wide (6)	Serratia (71) Klebsiella, Citrobacter, Proteus, Enterobacter, Providencia (65)	UTI	Simultaneous (3 yr)	Gm,tb,kn,am,cf,cb,st,su
Burn unit (7)	Klebsiella, Enterobacter, 3 other genera (NS)	Burn	Simultaneous (11 mo)	Tb,kn,ne
Hospital wide (8)	Klebsiella (66) E. coli, Enterobacter, Proteus (14)	UTI, wd, resp	Index case admitted with epidemic strain; remainder ∿ simultaneous (2 yr)	Gm,tb,kn,am,cf,cb,ch,su

*ICU = Intensive Care Unit; NS = not stated; UTI = urinary tract infection; wd = wound infection; resp = respiratory infection; gm = gentamicin; tb = tobramycin; kn = kanamycin; am = ampicillin; cf = cephalothin; cb = carbenicillin; st = streptomycin; ch = chloramphenicol; su = sulfonamide; ne = neomycin.

Epidemiology

The epidemiology of most plasmid outbreaks, specifically the reservoir for the resistance plasmids and where and when transfer of plasmids occurred, has been largely speculative. Transfer can occur in the gut, on skin, in urine and in the environment (e.g., in urine containers). In addition, relatively avirulent bacterial strains may serve as reservoirs for resistance. For example, gentamicin resistance in S. epidermidis or S. aureus may be mediated by identical plasmids which can pass between these two species in vitro and on human skin (10). Epidemiologic and plasmid studies suggest that gentamicin resistant S. epidermidis is frequently acquired by hospitalized patients and may represent an endemic, largely unrecognized reservoir for resistance in the more virulent S. aureus (11). Moreover, in our hospital, genetic re-arrangements of one epidemic gentamicin resistance plasmid have led to a family of four related resistance plasmids that are endemic in nosocomial Staphylococci (12).

Recognition

Plasmid outbreaks may be difficult to detect but should be sought through surveillance for the occurrence of multiple species or genera with identical or very similar multiple drug (or even just key drug) resistance patterns. If available, similar gel electrophoretic patterns of plasmid DNA could facilitate direction. Once recognized, plasmid epidemics are at present controlled much like single strain outbreaks. In the future, technologic refinements may facilitate more extensive epidemiologic investigation of plasmid and transposon resistance and allow more specific control measures.

Other multiple strain outbreaks. Occasionally common sources may become contaminated with several bacterial species, leading to common source spread of completely unrelated strains. Such outbreaks may go unrecognized unless one strain predominates or the strains or epidemiologic circumstances are very unusual.

CONTROL OF EPIDEMIC RESISTANCE (TABLE 3)

Table 3.
MEASURES FOR CONTROLLING EPIDEMIC RESISTANCE

Identify reservoirs
Colonized and infected patients
Environmental contamination ; common sources
Halt transmission
Improve handwashing and asepsis
Isolate colonized and infected patients
Eliminate any common source and disinfect environment
Separate susceptible patients
Treat colonized patients (topically or systemically)*
Close unit to new admissions
Modify host risk
Control antibiotic use
Use topical antimicrobials to forestall colonization*
Use bacterial interference to prevent (or elimiate) colonization*

*Experience with these approaches is limited and they should be considered experimental (see text).

Basic measures

Control of epidemics has traditionally involved efforts to shore up aseptic practices while an epidemiologic analysis of cases (and controls) is quickly undertaken to exclude common source exposures. Attempts to decrease transmission have usually involved isolating or cohorting infected and colonized patients. Identifying all colonized patients usually requires "culture surveys", which may be facilitated by use of selective (often antibiotic-containing) media. Susceptible patients, such as those with indwelling urinary catheters, have been physically separated to decrease the likelihood that personnel would passively carry pathogens from one patient or drainage bag to the next. In drastic situations, units have been closed to new admissions and/or antibiotics have been administered to patients colonized with multiply resistant bacteria (e.g., multiple drug resistant pneumococci (13)).

Antibiotic controls

In some outbreaks, antibiotic controls may help to restrict the spread of resistant bacteria. First, in closed, high density units like ICUs restricting antibiotic use may be important. In rare situations, antibiotic use has even been totally and successfully suspended. Second, antibiotic restriction may decrease selective pressures in some plasmid outbreaks. (There are also chemicals that "cure" bacterial plasmids in vitro but available agents are too toxic for use in humans.) Third, more careful dosing with aminoglycosides may decrease the chance that subinhibitory levels will select resistant subpopulations (due to spontaneous chromosomal mutations) particularly in sites which have large bacterial populations, like wounds or the respiratory tract. Fourth, control of antibiotics which select for sensitive precursors of resistant organisms (e.g., cephalosporins selecting for Pseudomonas) may be necessary.

Experimental approaches

Prophylaxis. Prophylactic topical antibiotics, used experimentally in one ICU to forestall pharyngeal colonization and pneumonia with P. aeruginosa appeared to work during limited studies, but when applied in the ICU in a continuous fashion, led to a compensatory increase in pneumonias caused by polymixin resistant bacilli. Similarly, use of the oral non-absorbable regimen of gentamicin-vancomycin-nystatin for "gut sterilization" on oncology units has led to significant problems with gentamicin resistant gram-negative bacilli. Even the ingenious use of prophylactic trimethoprim-sulfamethoxazole to give oncology patients "colonization resistance" (due to the preservation of anaerobic flora) has been thwarted by emergence of plasmid-mediated trimethoprim resistance among gram-negatives (14).

Bacterial interference. In the 1960's, attempts were made to use avirulent staphylococci to reduce colonization with epidemic strains. This form of bacterial interference to control epidemic colonization has been re-explored recently. In one study, pharyngeal implantation of alpha hemolytic streptococci successfully displaced resistant enteric organisms in infants in a neonatal ICU. In an outbreak, this approach was used with other measures to successfully control colonization of neonates by amikacin resistant Serratia and Klebsiella (15). However, this approach needsto be studied further before any conclusions can be made about its general applicability.

Intensive environmental decontamination. Another control measure from the past that is being re-investigated is disinfection of urinary catheter drainage bags. Earlier use of this method with formalin in drainage bottles ended when closed drainage systems were widely adopted. Nevertheless, closed systems cannot prevent contamination of collection bags indefinitely ; in 30 % of patients with initially sterile urine, contamination of the bag may precede bladder infection. In a recent study, disinfection of drainage bags with hydrogen peroxide forestalled the occurrence of urinary infection in patients with acute spinal injury. Since organisms may still ascend from the perineum around the catheter, disinfection of the bag may not prevent infection in the individual patient. However, bag disinfection may reduce reservoirs of contaminated urine in the hospital environment and warrants further study, including evaluation for emergence of disinfectant resistant strains.

CONTROL OF ENDEMIC RESISTANCE

Antibiotic resistance precautions

In our hospital, we have brought a variety of epidemic control measures to the endemic level and apply barrier nursing "antibiotic resistance precautions" (figure 2) aggressively to patients who are colonized or infected with aminoglycoside resistant gram-negative bacilli (16). In our experience, these precautions have markedly decreased the incidence of aminoglycoside resistant E. coli, Klebsiella and Enterobacter and probably have limited the extent of recurrent mini-epidemics of resistant Serratia (figure 3).

1. **Room – 1- or 2- bed room; no roommate with drainage tubes or Foley.**
2. **Gowns – not necessary.**
3. **Masks – not necessary.**
4. **Hands – must be washed on entering and leaving room.**
5. **Gloves – must be worn for all patient or secretion contact.**
6. **Articles – must have own urine measuring cup; rinse before and after use and leave Amphyl in bottom when not in use. Discard all secretions in plastic bags.**

Figure 2. "Antibiotic Resistance Precautions" placard (placed on door to patient's room or above bed).

In sharp contrast, the incidence of aminoglycoside resistant Pseudomonas does not appear to have been affected appreciably by barrier precautions and has more likely paralleled aminoglycoside use. In fact, we have frequently found that in individual patients P. aeruginosa became resistant in the face of aminoglycoside exposure (3). An update of our experience since 1977 through 1981 has confirmed our findings. Nonetheless, the incidence of multiply resistant gram-negative bacilli on our oncology unit has increased, possibly due to extensive use of oral nonabsorbable prophylactic antibiotics ; however, our barrier precautions appear to have contained the problem to this unit and also to have reduced cross-infection among these patients.

Multi-faceted approach

In our experience, the following multi-faceted approach can help control endemic aminoglycoside resistant gram-negative bacilli in acute care hospitals.

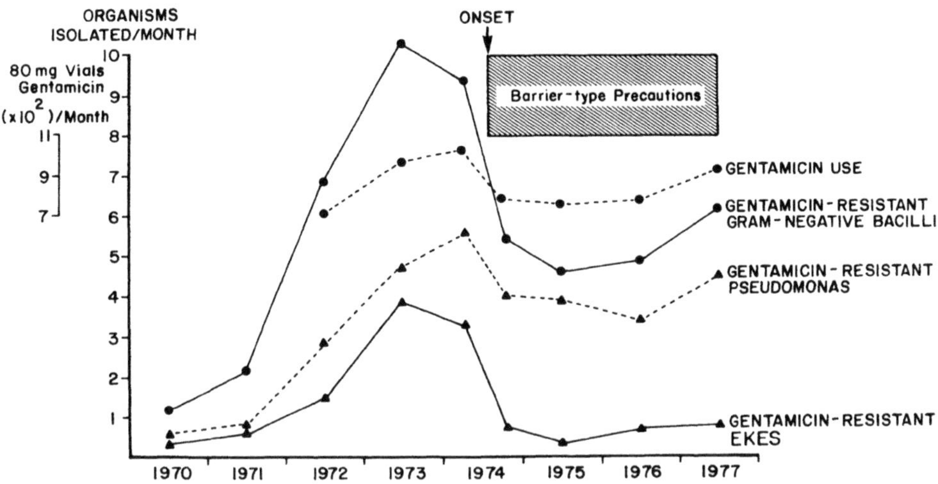

Figure 3. Gram-negative bacilli resistant to gentamicin and gentamicin usage at Michael Reese Medical Center, 1970-1977. (Reproduced with permission from Weinstein et al (16).) Data are plotted as the monthly average and the averages for the first seven and last five months of 1974 are plotted separately to demonstrate the effect of barrier-type precautions, which began in August 1974. EKES = Escherichia coli, Klebsiella pneumonia, Enterobacter species and Serratia species.

Antibiotic resistance precautions. These should be used for all patients who are colonized or infected with aminoglycoside resistant Enterobacteriaceae, methicillin resistant S. aureus and probably aminoglycoside resistant P. aeruginosa. These precautions should be extended to any patient who is colonized with other multiple drug resistant bacteria felt to be a problem in the hospital, expecially if the patient has significant drainage of secretions or requires intensive nursing care.

Admissions. Such precautions should be used while cultures are being processed from patients who are admitted (or readmitted) with a history of colonization or infection with multiply resistant organisms.

Transfers. Patients transferred from nursing homes or other hospitals should be evaluated for carriage of resistant bacilli. Certain patients, such as those with indwelling urinary catheters, may warrant precautions whil appropriate cultures are being processed if the epidemiologic background of the patient suggests high risk for resistance (e.g., residence in a nursing home known to have "resistance problems").
Aminoglycosides. Appropriate aminoglycoside usage and dosage should be assured to decrease selection of spontaneous mutations among P. aeruginosa and to a lesser extent among Enterobacteriaceae.
Other antibiotic controls. In certain specialty units such as ICUs, control of antibiotic usage (and in oncology units, limiting oral prophylactic regimens) may also help to control endemic resistance. However, several factors may limit the efficacy of antibiotic controls. First, use of one antibiotic may lead to cross resistance to others. We have seen aminoglycoside cross resistance, cross resistance to second and third generation cephalosporins after use of second generation drugs and plasmid colinkage of resistance. Next, sequential acquisition of bacterial resistance as antibiotics are rotated has been well described. Finally, if and when controls are lifted, resistant organisms that have remained in low numbers colonizing patients may reemerge.
Surveillance. Surveillance of patients and clinical laboratory results should be maintained to detect mini-epidemics of patients with similarly resistant organisms so that cross-infection or significant environmental reservoirs can be identified and controlled.

RESISTANCE PROBLEMS ON THE HORIZON

While aminoglycoside resistant gram-negative bacilli have been an essential concern of hospitals over the past ten years, a variety of new problems are emerging.

Resistant pneumococci have appeared in New Guinea and South Africa.

Methicillin-resistant S. aureus, a nosocomial problem in Europe in the 1960-1970's, have occurred with epidemic frequency in the community drug addict population of Detroit (USA), probably related to self-prescribing of cephalosporins to forestall "dirty injection" related infections (17). These strains have "spilled" into hospitals as admission of colonized and infected addicts has lead to extensive epidemics of nosocomial methicillin resistant S. aureus in that city.

As the incidence of infection with sensitive gram-negative bacilli has decreased in the oncology population due to use of oral nonabsorbable antibiotics coupled with empiric broad-spectrum systemic antibiotics, multiply resistant gram-postive bacteria, especially S. epidermidis and JK diphtheroids, have become increasingly frequent pathogens.

As noted above, the second and third generation cephalosporin drugs (and broad spectrum ureido-penicillins) appear to have a potential for inducing and/or selecting for resistance, particularly in Enterobacter species and this may well become the problem organism during the next few years.

As we increase our understanding of factors that control colonization with normal flora and that lead to overgrowth of resistant bacteria, new approaches to preventing colonization with nosocomial pathogens or blocking adherence of unwanted bacteria may emerge. Moreover, the growing interchange of resistant bacteria among nursing homes, community hospitals, tertiary care centers and high risk outpatient populations, such as drug addicts and chronically ill individuals, will continue to challenge our ability to work together.

REFERENCES

1. Stamm, W.E., Weinstein, R.A., Dixon, R.E. 1981. Comparison of endemic and epidemic nosocomial infections. Amer. J. Med. 70 : 393.
2. Schonfeld, H., Brockman, G.R.W., Hahn, F.E., eds. 1976. Antibiotics and chemotherapy. Vol. 20. Acquired resistance of micro-organisms to chemotherapeutic drugs. Basel : S. Karger.
3. Weinstein, R.A., Nathan, C., Gruensfelder, R., Kabins, S.A. 1980. Endemic aminoglycoside resistance in gram-negative bacilli : Epidemiology and mechanisms. J. Infect. Dis. 141 : 338.

4. Schaberg, D.R., Weinstein, R.A., Stamm, W.E. 1976. Epidemics of nosocomial urinary tract infection caused by multiply resistant gram-negative bacilli : Epidemiology and control. J. Infect. Dis 133 : 363.
5. Markowitz, S.M., Veazey, J.M., Macrina, F.L., Mayhall, C.G., Lamb, V.A. 1980. Sequential outbreaks of infection due to Klebsiella pneumoniae in a neonatal intensive care unit : Implication of a conjugative R plasmid. J. Infect. Dis. 142 : 106.
6. Tompkins, L.S., Plorde, J.J., Falkow, S. 1980. Molecular analysis of R factors from multiresistant nosocomial isolates. J. Infect. Dis. 141 : 625.
7. Elwell, L.P., Inamine, J.M., Minshew, B.H. 1978. Common plasmid specifying tobramycin resistance found in two enteric bacteria isolated from burn patients. Antimicrob. Agents Chemother. 13 : 312.
8. Sadowski, P.L., Peterson, B.C., Gerding, D.N., Cleary, P.P. 1979. Physical characterization of ten R plasmids obtained from an outbreak of nosocomial Klebsiella pneumoniae infections. Antimicrob. Agents Chemother. 15 : 616.
9. Rubens, C.E., Farrar, W.E., McGee, Z.E., Schaffner, W. 1981. Evolution of plasmid mediating resistance to multiple antimicrobial agents during a prolonged epidemic of nosocomial infections. J. Infect. Dis. 143 : 170.
10. Jaffe, H.W., Sweeney, H.M., Nathan, C., Weinstein, R.A., Kabins, S.A., Cohen, S. 1980. Identity and interspecific transfer of gentamicin-resistance plasmids in Staphylococcus aureus and Staphylococcus epidermidis. J. Infect. Dis. 141 : 738.
11. Weinstein, R.A., Kabins, S., Nathan, C., Sweeney, H., Jaffe, H., Cohen, S. 1982. Gentamicin-resistant staphylococci as hospital flora : Epidemiology and resistance plasmids. J. Infect. Dis. 145 : 374.
12. Jaffe, H., Sweeney, H., Weinstein, R.A., Nathan, C., Kabins, S., Cohen, S. 1982. Gentamicin-resistant staphylococci in hospital patients : Plasmid studies. Antimicrob. Agents Chemother. 21 : 773.
13. Koornhof, H.J., Jacobs, M.R., Ward, J.I., Appelbaum, P.C., Hallet, F.A. 1979. Therapy and control of antibiotic-resistant pneumococcal disease. Microbiology 286.
14. Jacoby, G.A. 1982. Perils of prophylaxis. N. Engl. J. Med. 306 : 43.
15. Cook, L.N., Davis, R.S., Stover, B.H. 1980. Outbreak of amikacin-resistant Enterobacteriaceae in an intensive care nursery. Pediatrics 65 : 264.
16. Weinstein, R.A., Kabins, S.A. 1981. Strategies for prevention and control of multiple drug-resistant nosocomial infections. Amer. J. Med. 70 : 449.
17. Saravolatz, L.D., Markowitz, N., Arking, L., Pohlod, D., Fisher, E. 1982. Methicillin-resistant Staphylococcus aureus. Epidemiologic observations during a community-acquired outbreak. Ann. Int. Med. 96 : 11.

COMPUTER MONITORING OF DRUG RESISTANCE IN THE HOSPITAL

R.P. MOUTON

INTRODUCTION

Specific resistance problems in a hospital are usually recognized by the bacteriologists responsible for laboratory reports. However, a gradually developing trend towards higher resistance frequencies in many species and for many antibiotics can only be found by time consuming review of all sensitivity test data or by computer. The signalling of certain multi-resistant patterns of given species can probably be done more reliably by a computerized system.

In The Netherlands uniform computer programs have been developed for many functions in several university hospitals, and include integral computer reporting by the microbiology laboratory. After introduction of the reporting system several years ago, the bacteriologists of three university hospitals devised several programs for "infection statistics", to retrieve epidemiological and sensitivity-test data from the data base. I should like to give a brief report on these programs which have now been operational for almost a year.

PROCEDURE FOR THE PROCESSING OF MICROBIOLOGICAL LABORATORY DATA

Each patient's specimen is numbered immediately after receipt, and his personal data together with data on the sample and type of request are introduced into the computer. After completion of the analysis, all data to be reported are also typed out for computer reporting (sometimes as a preliminary report), mostly in code. Printer terminals are located in all clinical departments.

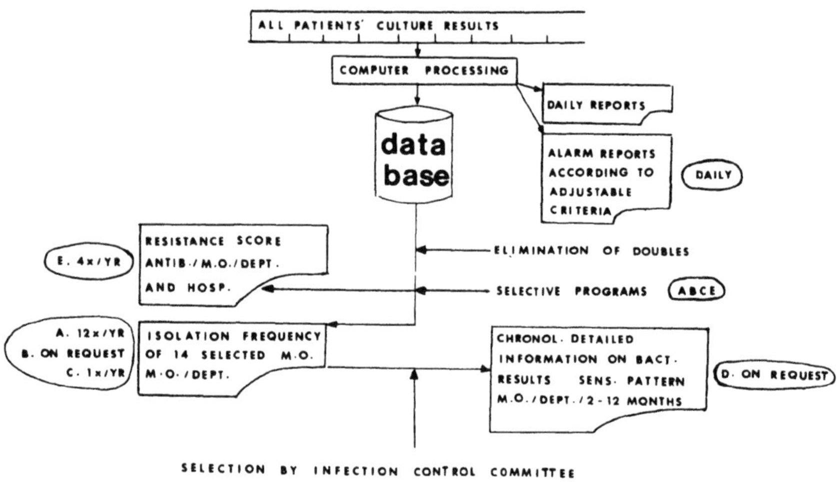

Fig. 1. Flow card for computerized infection control programs.

THE COMPUTERIZED INFECTION CONTROL PROGRAM

The programs we have at our disposal now and which will be discussed here, are limited to retrieval of laboratory data on the basis of specific data such as bacterial species, department, and sensitivity to one or more antibiotics. More general information on bacterial sensitivity development for surveillance purposes can also be obtained.

Cumulative data on clinical infections and their causes cannot be obtained by the present programs.

Fig. 1 shows a flow card representing the processing of laboratory data and the infection control program linked to it. The alarm system for multi-resistant bacteria can be programmed at will and prepares patient's reports for the infection control committee on the basis of data on resistance of one or more species to one or more antibiotics. At present this type of reporting takes place for:

a. gentamicin and/or tobramycin and/or amikacin resistance of Enterobacteriaceae and Pseudomonas aeruginosa;
b. kanamycin and/or methicillin resistance of Staphylococcus aureus; and
c. the isolation of Salmonella, Shigella or Serratia species.

However, the criteria can be adjusted.

The lay-out of programs A, B, and C presenting bacterial isolation data is given in Table 1. This type of reporting makes it possible to detect, either monthly or on demand, high isolation rates of one species in any department, as well as increases in these rates. Yearly print-outs should guarantee improved warning of slowly occurring increases of isolation rates.

It will be evident that isolation data alone are not sufficient to detect an increase of (cross) infections, because the number of isolations from one patient may have considerable effect on the total number of isolations registered. To eliminate this source of error duplicate isolations (e.g., same species, same sensitivity pattern, same patient's material) were counted as one. On the basis of the information given by this type of report, further details can be requested about a particular species in a given department. Program D (Table 2) was developed for this purpose. It presents the patient's personal data, the source of the isolate (e.g., sputum, blood etc.) and sensitivity-test results. Critical evaluation of these data may provide grounds for typing of strains; 8 positions on the computer print-out have been reserved for added data on typing. At every stage of our data assessment, decisions can be made on cross-infection analysis for a specific department.

Finally, data on resistance rates are generated quarterly (program E). Again we try to eliminate duplicates , but these cannot be completely avoided because small, possibly insignificant, differences in sensitivity patterns lead to double counts. The lay-out of the reports of program E is shown in Table 3. Because of the rather small number of strains per department, we are unable to draw conclusions about resistance-rate changes in one department. For the time being we must be content with the over-all data on the resistance rates for 17 antibiotics in our clinical and out-patient departments respectively.

Data on isolation rates have already contributed to the direction of the activities of the committee on infection control. However, no outbreaks have occurred and therefore the effectiveness of detection has not been put to the test yet. The alarm system on multi-resistant isolates has, however, an influence every day on the decisions taken by the infection-control committtee concerning the isolation of patients.

Our data on resistance rates are expected to serve as a basis for antibiotic policies in the future, but such data can only be properly evaluated over a longer period of time than our material covers at present.

INFECTIECOMMISSIE ACAD. ZIEKENH.LEIDEN

MAAND OVERZICHT DD: 12-10-1981

PERIODE: 01-08-1981 T/M 30-09-1981

AFD.	MND	STA	STRE	ENC	ESC	KLE	ENCL	- - - -
CARD	AUG	1	0	1	3	5	0	- - - -
	SEP	2	0	0	5	0	0	- - - -
CHIA	AUG	6	0	8	12	9	0	- - - -
	SEP	1	0	3	15	8	2	- - - -
CHIB	AUG	6	0	10	12	1	1	- - - -
	SEP	9	0	5	9	3	3	- - - -
CHID	AUG	10	0	2	11	2	0	- - - -
	SEP	3	0	2	5	4	2	- - - -
CHKL	AUG	2	0	6	7	1	4	- - - -
	SEP	4	1	5	5	2	4	- - - -
⋮	⋮	⋮	⋮	⋮	⋮	⋮	⋮	
VRV	AUG	1	0	3	6	0	1	- - - -
	SEP	1	0	1	6	2	0	- - - -
REST	AUG	97	6	26	161	33	7	- - - -
	SEP	79	12	27	182	40	9	- - - -
TOT.	AUG	241	10	122	405	102	27	- - - -
	SEP	198	16	95	381	104	39	- - - -

Table 1. Lay-out of monthly report on isolation rates of 14 bacterial species in 30 hospital departments.
AFD: department; MND: month; STA: Staphylococcus aureus; STR: Streptococcus group A; ENC: Enterococcus; ESC: Escherichia sp.; KLE: Klebsiella sp.;
ENCL: Enterobacter cloacae.
REST: combined out-patient departments.

INFECTIECOMMISSIE ACAD. ZIEKENH.LEIDEN BLZ 1

OVERZICHT D : 1 ISOLAATTYPE PER AFDELING DD: 07-12-1981

PERIODE: 01-10-1981 T/M 07-12-1981

AFDELING:KIND (GROEP)
ISOLAAT :STAPHYLOCOCCUS AUREUS

PAT.NR.	PATIENTNAAM	M/V	MONNR.		MA	MATDAT	AFD.	OPNDAT	PES	CLX	AMP	TIC	CEF	CFM	ERY	CHL	TET	KAN	GEN	TOB
8449567	AS....	M	142342	U	UK	011081	KINB	011081#	S	S			S		S	S	S	S	S	
4545277	CA...	M	143070	H	UN	071081	KINB	051081#	R	S			S		S	S	S	S	S	
8392511	BE...	M	143091	I	LI	071081	KINB	071081	R	S			S		S	S	S	S	S	
5531715	WI..	M	144326	Y	UN	151081	KINB	141081#	R	S			S		S	S	S	S	S	
4318673	KU..	M	147050	B	UN	031181	KINB	031181#	R	S			S		S	S	I	S	S	
4318673	KU..	M	147050	B	UN	031181	KINB	031181#	R	S			S		S	I	I	S	S	
4316496	SM..	V	148379	M	UN	111181	KINB	111181#	R	S			S		S	S	S	S	S	
1561501	LA.....	M	148818	Y	UN	131181	KINB	061181#	R	S			S		S	S	S	S	S	

Table 2. Lay-out of specified data on isolation of one species in one department. The survey period is two months now, but will be made adjustable. Sensitivity test data are given on the right. MA: type of specimen; MATDAT: date of specimen; OPNDAT: date of hospitalization.

```
INFECTIECOMMISSIE ACAD. ZIEKENH.LEIDEN
**************************************************
KWARTAALOVERZICHT RESISTENTIESPECTRA PER AFD.
**************************************************
PERIODE: 01-07-1981 T/M 30-09-1981
**********************************
                              DD: 15-01-1982
   ISOLAAT :ESC  (GROEP)
```

AFD.		PEN	AMP	TIC	CEF	CFM	- - - -
CARD	T	13	13	13	12	13	- - - -
13	%U	0	7	0	0	0	- - - -
	%S	0	69	84	83	100	- - - -
	%I	0	23	7	16	0	- - - -
	%R	100	0	7	0	0	- - - -
CHIA	T	37	37	37	25	37	- - - -
37	%U	0	0	0	4	0	- - - -
	%S	0	56	94	76	100	- - - -
	%I	2	40	2	20	0	- - - -
	%R	97	2	2	0	0	- - - -
	⋮	⋮	⋮	⋮	⋮	⋮	
VRV	T	18	18	18	13	18	- - - -
18	%U	0	5	0	0	0	- - - -
	%S	0	61	100	84	100	- - - -
	%I	0	33	0	15	0	- - - -
	%R	100	0	0	0	0	- - - -
REST	T	514	513	511	477	511	- - - -
514	%U	0	0	0	2	2	- - - -
	%S	0	57	79	66	88	- - - -
	%I	1	21	1	28	9	- - - -
	%R	98	20	18	2	0	- - - -
TOT.	T	1166	1165	1162	923	1161	- - - -
1166	%U	0	0	0	3	2	- - - -
	%S	0	56	78	64	87	- - - -
	%I	0	21	1	28	8	- - - -
	%R	99	21	19	3	1	- - - -

Table 3. Lay-out of quarterly report on resistance rates of eight bacterial species in 30 clinical departments and the combined out-patient departments (REST). AFD: department; T: total number of strains per department; %R: per cent resistant strains; %I: per cent intermediate strains; %S: per cent sensitive strains; %U: per cent of strains sensitive at the urinary concentration level; ESC: Escherichia coli; PEN, AMP, TIC, CEF, CFM: abbreviations for antibiotics.

DISCUSSION EDITED BY R.P. MOUTON

Thompson: You recommend that gloves be worn for all contacts with a patient, but this hampers physical examination. And since the stethoscope is a potential vehicle for spreading organisms, would you advocate a separate stethoscope for each patient?

Weinstein: If surgeons can handle delicate tissue wearing tight gloves, we feel we should be able to palpate or percuss with gloves on. You may not agree, but we do it. We have not made disinfection of stethoscopes mandatory; we have cultured bacteria from stethoscopes but have not found them to be a particular problem with respect to Gram-negatives, although we realize this is possible.

van der Meer: I am always worried by the fact that most of the antibiotics we use appear in the urine in high concentration. To prevent selective pressure of these antibiotics on the nosocomial flora, perhaps we should look for ways to inactivate these drugs in the urine. What is your opinion about this?

Weinstein: It is an interesting thought.

Mouton: You mentioned that cross-infection was responsible for the spread of resistant bacteria in about 40% of the cases, 25% being due to antibiotic pressure, about 20% acquired from the community, and about 20% from other sources. How can you separate these specific sources? Doesn't selection by antiboitc pressure have a strong influence on the acquisition of bacteria from other sources? Did you not find that a combination of factors could play a role?

Weinstein: Cases of resistance due to antibiotic pressure were largely those where we found sensitive organisms first, and resistant organisms of the same serotype later on. Cross-infections represented the time-space clusters; often more than one factor was operative in a patient.

Jackson: Would you share your data on the carrier state for Enterobacteriaceae with us? You said that personnel are rarely persistent carriers of these micro-organisms, in contrast to staphylococci. Yet in the epidemics that have been studied, gut colonization of the patients was an early and highly prevalent phenomenon. I don't know about the personnel. Have you studied the gut colonization of personnel?

Weinstein: We have looked at this in different ways. First, isolates from about 20 pseudomonas outbreaks were sent for typing to the Center for Disease Control. In a number of these cases, personnel were gut carriers of pseudomonas of the same serotype involved in an outbreak, but control of the outbreak occurred without removal of these persons from the hospital; in some cases the serotypes were different. In a prospective study in our intensive-care unit, we looked at hand carriage of pseudomonas. One may assume this to be an intermediate step in cross-infection. Out of many personnel, we found one nurse who was a persistent carrier of the same serotype of pseudomonas over a four-week period, but we found no evidence for transmission of the nurse's organism. Well-documented outbreaks in which a personnel carrier of resistant Gram-negative organisms has been implicated, are scarce.

Goldmann: The Center for Disease Control in the U.S. has been saying for a decade that we should do surveilance for true infections and not just for bacteria. It is very important not to rely only on routine screening of cultures to detect the extent of the spread of the organism. We used selective media containing the antibiotic that we were interested in, for instance gentamicin. We found that in a group of cytstic fibrosis patients producing sputum with pseudomonas in it, less than 1% of the organisms were resistant to the aminoglycosides and 99% or more of the flora in one patient may be sensitive; by only using routine methods you miss the resistant ones. Treatment with the aminoglycoside then selects the resistant strain and a new reservoir for the further spread of resistance is created. Would you agree, Dr. Weinstein, that the use of selective media to assess the extent of the spread of resistance can be useful epidemiologically?

Weinstein: A prospective study of this kind is being analysed now, but I cannot give you an answer yet. Secondly, we do have a computer program similar to the one described, but due to organizational and technical problems we have never been able to use the program on an ongoing day-to-day basis. However, it has been very helpful for retrospective studies, the analysis of trends, and in the making of policy decisions. As an actual day-to-day system we have not had much luck with it.

Mouton: I agree that these data can only be used on a retrospective basis with one exception, which is the immediate reporting of resistant strains. By using the program there is less risk of missing patients that should be isolated or otherwise taken care of because they carry resistant strains.

OCCURRENCE OF INFECTIONS AND ANTIBIOTIC PROPHYLAXIS IN NON-SURGICAL PATIENTS

P.J. VAN DEN BROEK and W.E. FIBBE

INTRODUCTION

The present paper concerns the occurrence and prophylaxis of hospital infections in patients whose humoral and/or cellular immunity is compromised. Of all the patients who are candidates for any kind of antibiotic prophylaxis not related to surgical treatment (Table I), this group runs the highest risk of becoming infected in the hospital. Because antibiotic prophylaxis in these patients cannot be evaluated apart from the other preventive measures taken concomitantly, prophylaxis will be discussed as a whole.

Table I.

ANTIMICROBIAL PROPHYLAXIS IN NON-SURGICAL PATIENTS

Endocarditis
Rheumatic fever
Meningococcal meningitis
Recurrent urinary-tract infections
Recurrent erysipelas
Pneumocystis carinii
Tuberculosis
Antimicrobial decontamination of the gut
Traveler's diarrhoea

A hospital infection is defined as an infection that is known to have originated in the hospital, taking into account the incubation time for that particular kind of infection. Hospital infections can be divided into exogenous and endogenous infections (Fig. 1). The exogenous hospital infections arise directly from contamination in the hospital. An endogenous infection in the strict sense of the term originates from the patient's own microbial flora, which is present on admission. It must be kept in mind that many micro-organisms acquired in the hospital colonize before they give rise to an infection at some later time (1-4). This kind of infection is called an endogenous infection in the broader sense of the term.

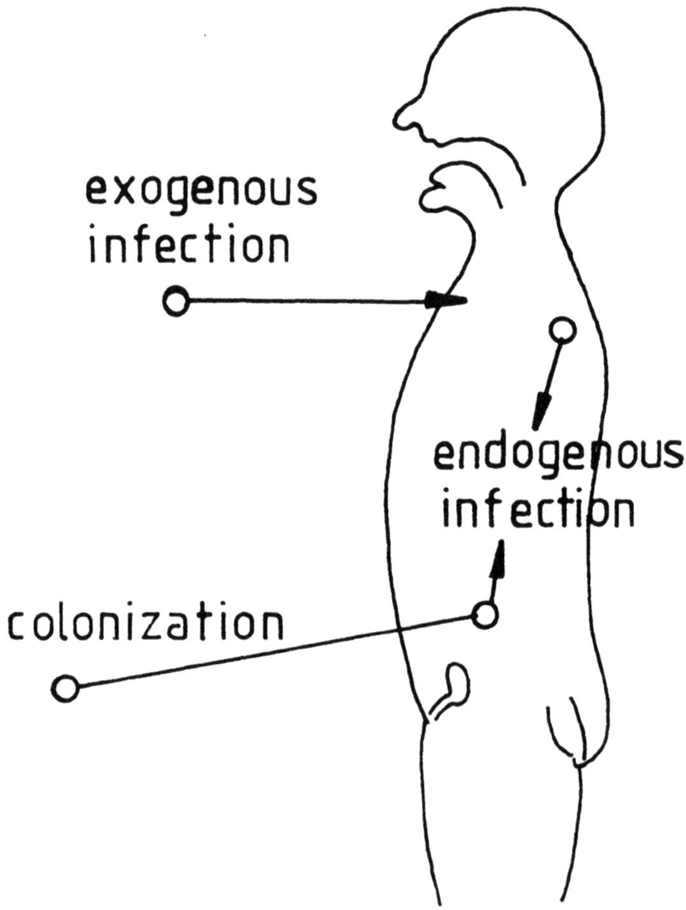

Fig. 1. Schematic representation of the concept of exogenous and endogenous hospital infections.

The present paper is limited to bacterial and fungal infections; protozoal and helminthic infections will only be mentioned incidentally. The prevention of viral infections, although of great importance, is beyond the scope of this paper.

OCCURRENCE

Only some aspects of the occurrence of hospital infections in immuno-compromised patients will be mentioned, i.e., where relevant for the discussion of the prevention of infections. More extensive information can be found in the papers of L.S. Young, D.A. Goldman, and R.H. Rubin in this volume, as well as in many review articles (5-9).

Granulocytopenia is a major risk factor and there is a distinct relationship between the occurrence of infections and the degree of granulocytopenia: most of the infections occur when the number of granulocytes is below 0.1×10^9 1 (10,11). The nature of the infections is related to the nature of the impairment of the host defense (Table II). Granulocytopenia is chiefly associated with bacterial and fungal infections.

In 1981 we evaluated 70 granulocytopenic episodes (number of granulocytes lower than $0.5 \times 10^9/1$) accompanied by fever (temperature higher than 38°C, measured in the axilla) in 60 patients. The characteristics of these patients are given in Table III. During these 70 granulocytopenic episodes, 22 minor and 59 major bacteriologically or clinically documented infections were observed. Details of the infections are given in Tables IV and V. The number of fungal infections is low, i.e., 2 (3.3% in 60 patients), compared with the data in the literature (i.e., 15%) (12,13). Infection was the definite or possible cause of death in 16 of the 26 fatal cases (60%). Half of these 16 patients were refractory to the therapy applied for the haematological malignancy, and three others were admitted with the infection and died within 24 hours, either before therapy could be instituted or despite the institution of adequate antimicrobial therapy.

Table II. HOST RESISTANCE AND INFECTION

HOST RESISTANCE	HOST RESITANCE DISTURBED BY	MOST IMPORTANT PATHOGENS
1) Surface		
Mechanical barrier	wounds, foreign bodies, haematoma, ischaemia, catheters, instrumentation	(colonizing) bacteria
Secretional barrier		
sebum, sweat,		
mucus,	cystic fibrosis, parasympathiolytic drugs,	
gastric acid,	antacids, H2-receptor blocking drugs, vagotomy, gastrectomy	Salmonella species, Shigella species
lysozyme,		
immunoglobulins	hypogammaglobulinaemia, selective IgA deficiency	encapsulated bacteria; Giardia lamblia
Elimination by motility		
cilia	immotile cilia syndrome, alcoholism, smoking	
cough	anaesthesia, morphinomimetic drugs	
peristalsis	parasympathicolytic and morphinomimetic drugs, obstruction	(colonizing) bacteria
micturition	parasympathiocolytic drugs, obstruction	
desquamation		
2) Humoral defence		
Aspecific		
lysozyme		
lactoferrin		
complement	primary and secondary deficiencies: C3/C5	encapsulated bacteria, Gram-negative bacteria
	C6, 7 and 8	Neisseria spp.
Specific		
antibodies	hypogammaglobulinaemia	encapsulated bacteria; Giardia lamblia
3) Cellular defence		
Phagocytosis by		
granulocytes, monocytes/macro-phages	quantitative defects (myelosuppression), qualitative defects (e.g., congenital defects, effects of drugs, diabetes, cirrhosis)	bacteria (especially staphylococci and Gram-negative bacteria), fungi
Cell-mediated immunity		
T lymphocytes + macrophages	quantitative and qualitative defects (primary immunodeficiency, immunosuppressive drugs	obligate and facultative

Table III.

RELEVANT CHARACTERISTICS OF 60 PATIENTS WITH GRANULOCYTOPENIA AND FEVER

Number of granulocytopenic episodes	70	
Number of males	33	
Number of females	27	
age (mean + range)	40.8	(16-77)
Number of days with less than $0.5 \times 10^9/l$ granulocytes	1766	
median (interquartile range)	24	(14-32)
Number of days with less than $0.1 \times 10^9/l$ granulocytes	1233	
median (interquartile range)	16	(7-24)
Haematological status	patients	episodes
diagnosis: acute non-lymphocytic leukaemia	40	49
acute lymphocytic leukaemia	5	5
aplastic anaemia	6	7
lymphoma	6	6
blast crisis chronic myeloid leukaemia	3	3
prognosis: first granulocytopenic episode	31	
second and subsequent granulocytopenic episode	39	
Preventive measures		
protective isolation		
simple	44	
advanced	19	
none	7	
antimicrobial decontamination		
pad	34	
pad + cotrim	2	
cotrim	4	

Table IV.

INFECTIONS IN 70 GRANULOCYTOPENIC EPISODES WITH FEVER

Minor infections	22	
of the oropharynx		13
cellulitis		2
hydradenitis		1
others		6
Major infections	59	
with septicaemia due to Gram-positive micro-organisms		16
with septicaemia due to Gram-negative micro-organisms		18
candidaemia		1
without septicaemia		
digestive tract		4
pneumonia		16
soft tissues		14

Table V.

SOURCES OF MICRO-ORGANISMS CAUSING SEPTICAEMIA

	Gram-negative micro-organisms	Gram-positive micro-organisms
Lung	2	2
Digestive tract	10	3
Oropharynx	2	0
Intravenous catheter	0	8
Unknown	4	3

PREVENTION

The prevention of infections in hospitalized patients must be based primarily on a policy aiming to avoid as much as possible any impairment of the host defense and the ecological balance of the patient's microbial flora. The possible value of any treatment must be weighed in terms of its effect on the host's resistance to infections, and when possible alternatives with less deleterious effects on the host defense must be evaluated. This holds for all procedures; for example, urinary catheters should only be used if urgently needed, and repetition of venapuncture should be preferred to leaving an intravenous catheter in situ to drain blood or administer drugs. The fact that among the 19 infections we observed during 1981 in patients nursed in laminar air flow rooms, 8 originated from intravenous cathethers, clearly illustrates the problems created by these catheters. In 2 of the 8 cases of septicaemia, endocarditis was suspected because the blood cultures continued to be positive after removal of the catheter, and one patient died due to secondary localization in the brain and meninges (14).

Concerning the choice of antimicrobial therapy for an infection, the extent to which a given antibiotic will influence the patient's microbial flora must be taken into account. Great reserve should be exercised in the use of antibiotics, because of the unequivocal relationship between this form of treatment, the selection of multiply resistant micro-organisms (15), and the occurrence of secondary infections with such micro-organisms and fungi (16,17). Furthermore, the superfluous use of antibiotics also has an undesirable effect on the susceptibility to antibiotics of the pathogenic micro-organisms in the hospital (18), and consideration must be given to the possibility of drug toxicity and the difficulties antibiotics create for bacteriological diagnosis (19).

However, the question is whether it is possible to be sparing with antimicrobial agents in immuno-compromised patients. In most hospitals today, the general approach in granulocytopenic patients is to administer antibiotics whenever fever occurs that cannot be ascribed to some other cause such as a blood transfusion, a viral infection, or a drug reaction. This policy is based on the opinion that it is often very difficult to diagnose an infection in granulocytopenic patients, and that the course of infections that are not recognized and therefore are not treated, is rapidly fatal. Our approach to the treatment of the granulocytopenic patients with fever -- which pays more attention to the risks involved in the use of antibiotics -- is shown in Fig. 2.

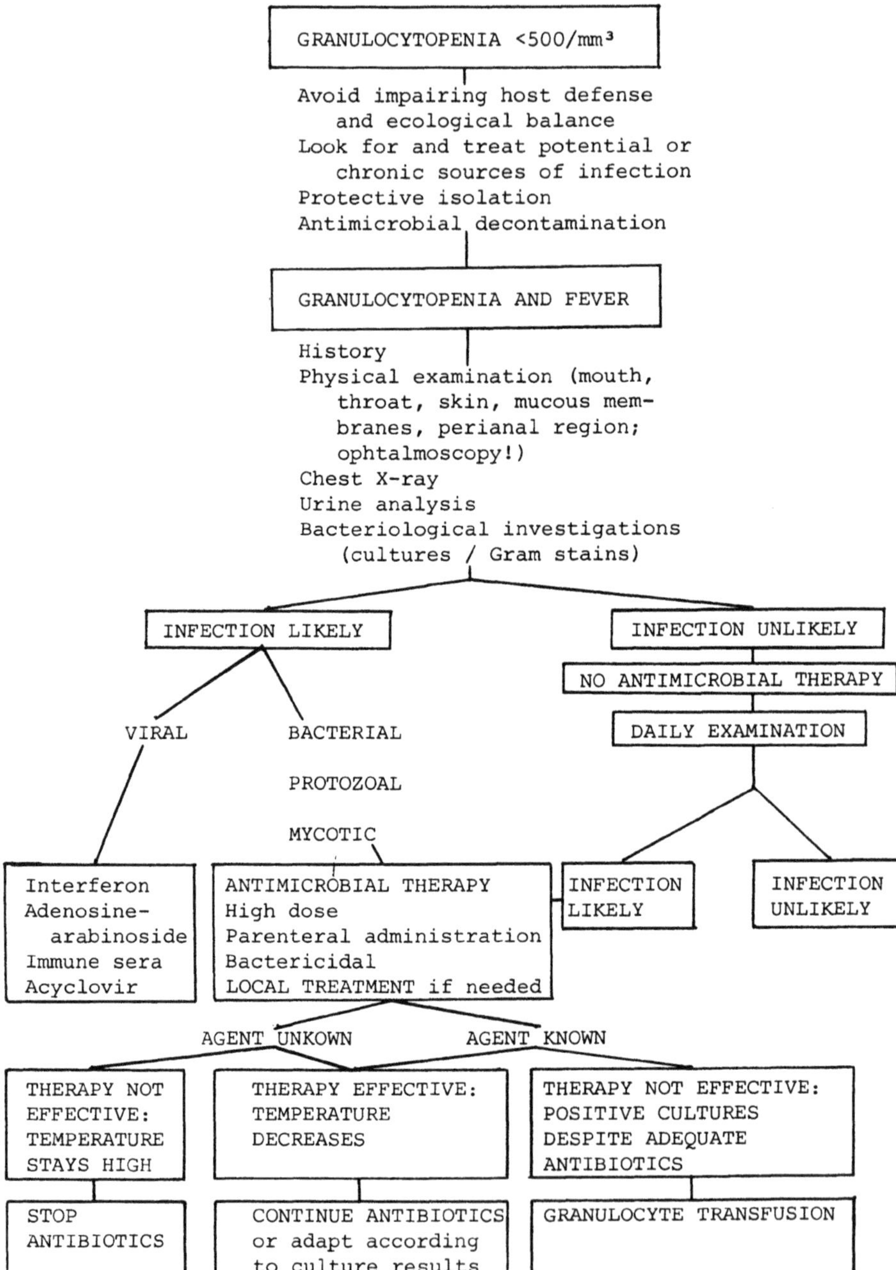

Fig. 2. The low-antibiotic approach to the granulocytopenic patient with fever.

When a granulocytopenic patient runs a fever, his history should be taken and he should be examined carefully, with special attention to the mucous membranes and the skin. Radiographs of the chest and the sinusses should be made and a urine analysis and bacteriological investigations should be performed. The results will usually indicate whether an infection is likely or not. If infection is unlikely, antimicrobial therapy should not be instituted. The patient should be kept under close observation and examined at least once daily. If an infection becomes probable, antimicrobial therapy is started immediately. The choice of antibiotic depends on the nature of the infection (20). If the therapy is not effective and the causative agent remains unknown, therapy should be stopped and the diagnostic procedures repeated. If the causative agent is known and the therapy is not effective despite being adequate as to in vitro sensitivity, dosage, and route of administration, granulocyte transfusions can be given.

The second principle of infection prevention in immunocompromised patients or patients expected to become immunocompromised in the near future, is to look for potential or chronic sources of infection and to treat these sources, if possible before the institution of any therapy that will further compromise the host defense. Possible sources of infection are listed in Table VI, as well as the diagnostic methods used to detect these sources and indications for their elimination.

Table VI.

DIAGNOSIS AND HANDLING OF POTENTIAL SOURCES AND CHRONIC SITES OF INFECTION

Source / site	Diagnosis	Treatment
Carious teeth	physical examination	dental care
Root granuloma	X-ray	dental care
(Chronic) sinusitis	X-ray; sinus puncture	nose drops, flushing; eventualy antibiotics
(Asymptomatic) urinary-tract infection	urological examination	depends on underlying disease
Phimosis	physical examination	circumcision
Anal fissure	physical examination	delation of anus; laxative diet
(Recurrent) boils	history / physical examination	antiseptic soap, and disinfective ointment for the nose
Ingrowing toenail	physical examination	excision
Carrier state of		
S. aureus	history / culture of nose	antiseptic soap, and disinfective ointment for the nose
Salmonella spp.	culture of faeces	cholecystectomy, cotrimoxazole
Strept. pneumoniae	culture of throat	penicillin G
Strongyloides stercoralis	parasite in faeces or duodenal fluid	thiabendazole
Entamoeba histolytica	cysts, trophozoites in faeces, rectal biopsy; serology	metronidazole; emetine

In the examination of the patient, special attention should be paid to the teeth, the skin, the external genitalia, and the perianal region. Radiography of the teeth and sinusses should be made routinely. A bacteriological inventory is performed, including cultures of materials from the throat, the nose, the perineum, and samples of urine and faeces, to detect asymptomatic bacteriuria and carrier states of Staphylococcus aureus, Salmonella spp., and Streptococcus pneumoniae. In patients who have lived in (sub)tropical countries, the faeces must also be investigated for the presence of eggs, cysts, or vegetative forms of Entamoeba histolytica and Strongyloides stercoralis. If any possible source of infection or chronic infection is diagnosed, treatment should be started immediately.

The third principle of prevention is assessment of the extent to which a particular patient can be expected to benefit from special measures, such as protective isolation, decontamination, granulocyte transfusions, vaccination, or antimicrobial prophylaxis aimed at a specific micro-organism, e.g. Mycobacterium tuberculosis or Pneumocystis carinii. Granulocyte transfusions are not recommended for prophylactic use, because the risks outweigh the benefits (21). All patiens who have undergone splenectomy and patients with sickle-cell anaemia should be vaccinated with pneumococcal vaccine, because these patients run a high risk of acquiring severe pneumococcal infection. Vaccination against Pseudomonas aeruginosa lowers the rate of infection with this micro-organism, but the protection does not last long. This and the side effects, make this vaccination only of value for prophylaxis for short duration, e.g., patients with burns. Vaccination against endotoxins of Gram-negative bacilli is still Utopian, although much work is being done in this field (22). Prophylaxis with isoniazide for tuberculosis should be given to any patient who has suffered from tuberculosis in the past and has or can be expected to develop impaired cell-mediated immunity. Prophylaxis with cotrimoxazole for Pneumocystis carinii, which was introduced by Hughes (23), proved to be an effective method to prevent such infections as long as the drugs are taken. This prophylaxis is indicated for patients at relatively high risk with respect to Pneumocystis carinii pneumonia, for instance children with acute lymphocytic leukaemia.

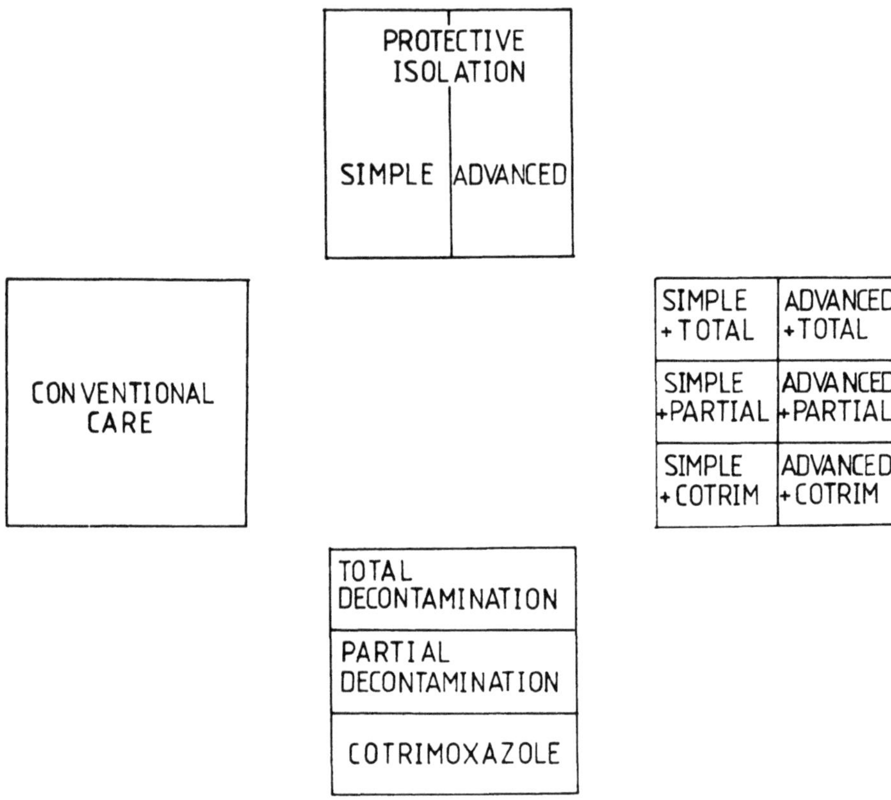

Fig. 3a. Various possibilities for protective isolation and antimicrobial decontamination.

The various alternatives to the use of protective isolation and antimicrobial decontamination alone or together, are shown in Fig. 3a.

Protective isolation

Many varieties of protective isolation are available, ranging from nursing the patient in a simple single-bed room, with or without a sluice or with or without a ventilation system, to laminar air flow rooms and plastic tent isolators. Protective isolation aims to interrupt the routes of contamination to the patient who is at risk with respect to acquiring a hospital infection. Contamination of the patient can take place via the air and direct or indirect contact. To avoid contamination via the air, the patient is nursed separated from other patients in the hospital. To cut off contamination by direct contact, each person who comes into contact with the patient has to take precautionary measures such as hand washing and wearing a gown used only for that patient. Contamination by indirect contact is prevented by the use of sterile materials for nursing of the patient. Since the patient's food is a major source of contamination, it should have a low bacterial content, which can be achieved by cooking all food well and serving it immediately and as hot as possible.

Decontamination

Protective isolation is designed to deal with exogenous infections and by controlling the colonization of the patient with endogenous infections in the broader sense of the term. However, the patient takes his own bacterial flora with him into the protective isolation, and this bacterial flora can also be a source of infections, the most important source being the digestive tract, from the mouth to the anus. The chance of becoming infected would seem to be much smaller if this bacterial flora were eliminated or suppressed. This is indeed the case in germ-free animals, which can survive granulocytopenia without serious infectious problems (24). This led to the development of several methods to eliminate or suppress the patient's bacterial flora. Total decontamination aims at the elimination of all of the micro-organisms borne by the patient. Attempts have been made to achieve this state by the administration of non-absorbable oral antibiotics, sometimes together with topically applied antibiotics and antiseptics (25,26), but it proved impossible to achieve a germ-free state in this way (27,28). This led to the design of an elaborate rotating scheme with multiple antibiotics that are orally absorbable or are even administered systemically (29). This method too failed to establish a germ-free state.

Partial or selective decontamination does not affect the anaerobic micro-organisms in the digestive tract. Only the aerobic Gram-negative micro-organisms are eliminated. This is useful, because anaerobic bacteria diminish the colonization of the digestive tract by aerobic Gram-negative bacteria: much higher numbers of micro-organisms are needed to colonize the gut in the presence than in the absence of the anaerobic bacteria (30). This phenomenon is called colonization resistance.

Unlike total decontamination, which is very difficult to achieve, a state of partial decontamination can be reached and maintained relatively easily.

Decontamination with cotrimoxazole

Decontamination with cotrimoxazole is not merely decontamination but also systemic antibiotic prophylaxis, because cotrimoxazole is absorbed in the gut. This form of prophylaxis takes into account the principle of colonization resistance, since cotrimoxazole has no effect on the anaerobic micro-organisms in the digestive tract (31), but eliminates or suppresses the aerobic Gram-negative bacteria.

Effectiveness of protective isolation, decontamination, and a combination of the two procedures

The decision whether to stick to a particular way of treating immunocompromised patients or to change to another regimen, must be based on knowledge about the effectiveness of each regimen compared with that of other regimens, the degree to which a particular regimen is tolerated by the patients, the patient's compliance, the unfavourable effects of the various regimens, and the costs involved.

The effectiveness of the various procedures is assessed on the basis of the following criteria:

1) The infection rate, i.e., the percentage of patients with an infection; this is calculated with the equation:

$$\frac{\text{number of infections x 100}}{\text{number of patients}}.$$

2) The number of infections per 1000 days at risk, i.e., the number of days on which the number of granulocytes was lower than $0.5 \times 10^9/l$; this is calculated with the equation:

$$\frac{\text{number of infections x 1000}}{\text{days at risk}}.$$

This figure permits a cautious comparison of the results of different investigators.

3) The therapeutic gain, i.e., the difference between the infection rates of the two groups compared in a controlled clinical trial. The 95% confidence limits were estimated (32). These 95% confidence limits mean that we can be 95% certain that the true difference between the two methods lies between the two limits, which in turn gives an idea of the therapeutic gain to be expected from switching from method one to another.

4) The conclusion drawn by the investigators of a particular method as to the effectiveness of that method.

It was not possible to apply all of these criteria in all the investigations discussed here, because essential information was lacking in many publications.

Effectiveness of protective isolation

To achieve successful protective isolation, separation of the patient from the hospital environment must be combined with measures pertaining to nursing care and the provision of food with a low bacterial content. If any of these measures is neglected, protective isolation will be less effective or fail. Lowbury et al. (33) and Cason et al. (34) investigated the effect of different methods of protective isolation on colononization by Staphylococcus aureus, Pseudomonas aeruginosa, and enterobacteriaceae in patients with burns. Except for separation of the patient from the hospital environment, almost no further measures were taken. The results of these investigations are shown in Table VII. The rate of colonization with S. aureus was only reduced slightly when the patient was nursed in a completely closed plastic tent. Colonization with Ps. aeruginosa was diminished when direct contact with the patient was made impossible, and colonization with enterobacteriaceae was not influenced by any of the methods of protective isolation investigated.

Table VII.

COMPARISON OF DIFFERENT METHODS OF PROTECTIVE ISOLATION IN PATIENTS WITH BURNS

Mode of hospitalization	Colonization of the patient		
	S. aureus	Ps. aeruginosa	Entero-bacteriaceae
Open ward	+++	+++	n.d.
1- or 2-bed room	+++	+++	n.d.
1- or 2-bed room + ventilation	+++	+++	n.d.
Air curtain	+++	+++	+++
Plastic isolator open top	+++	+	+++
Plastic isolator fully closed	++	+	+++

n.d. = is not done

Another example of the ineffectiveness of protective isolation when all of the measures concerning separation, handling, and food are not taken, is given by Lidwell and Towers (35): the acquisition of S. aureus and Gram-negative species was the same for patients nursed in laminar air flow rooms and in an open ward. When separation is combined with measures related to handling of the patients, a real decrease in colonization by S. aureus and Ps. aeruginosa is observed (36,37). Winner et al. (36) observed a decrease not only in the colonization rate, but also in the number of infections in the patients nursed in protective isolation compared with those nursed in an open ward.

The positive effect of protective isolation (laminar airflow rooms) on the prevention of infections in granulocytopenic patients was also shown by Yates and Holland (38) and Dietrich et al. (39). Yates and Holland (38) reported that no infections occurred after the 23rd day in the isolated patients, whereas infections continued to occur in non-isolated patients. The difference in the number of infections of the respiratory tract was particulary marked.

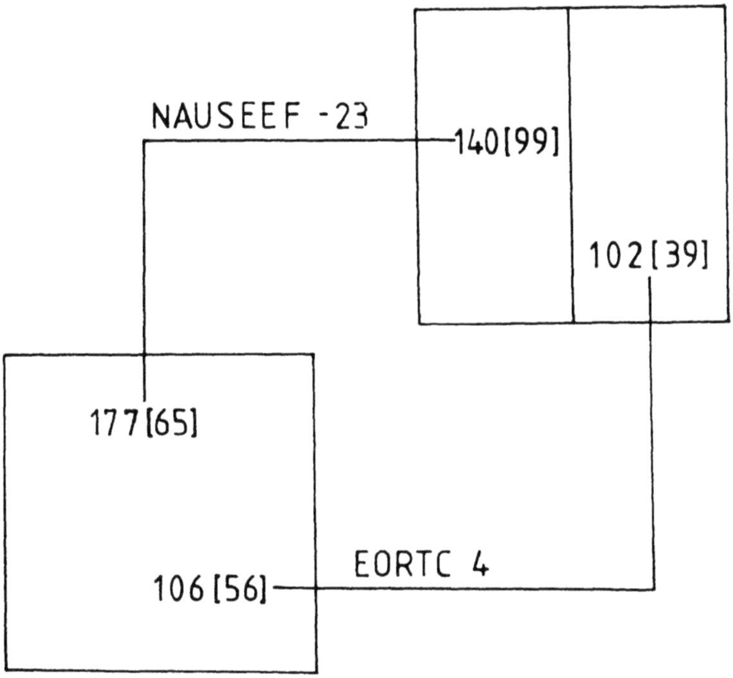

Fig. 3b. The effectiveness of protective isolation compared with standard care. In Fig. 3, b-e, the infection rate is given in the relevant area of the scheme. The number of infections per 1000 days at risk is given in parentheses , The difference between the infection rates is shown after the author's name where it was possible to calculate this parameter; where it was possible to calculate 95% confidence limits the values are given in parentheses ().

Dietrich et al. (39)(Fig. 3b) reported 39 infections per 1000 days at risk in isolated patients (laminar airflow rooms) as against 56 infections in non-isolated patients. Here, too, there was a striking difference in the number of infections of the respiratory tract. Nauseef and Maki (40) reported no difference in the acquisition of S. aureus and Ps. aeruginosa between patients nursed in single-bed rooms and with simple nursing-care measures and patients nursed in two-bed rooms with conventional care. However, the rate of acquisition of micro-organisms in these patients is low (about 4%) when compared with the 60% reported by Schmipff et al. (4); thus, a further reduction could not be accomplished in this study. The number of infections was 99 per 1000 days at risk for the isolated and 65 for the non-isolated patients (Fig. 3b).

Three conclusions can be drawn from these publications: 1) protective isolation must comprise separation combined with measures concerning handling of the patient and the food; 2) protective isolation reduces the rate of colonization and the rate of infections acquired in the hospital; and 3) it is impossible to assess the relative effectiveness of each of the methods of protective isolation.

Effectiveness of decontamination

Total decontamination

In two studies (25,26) the effect of total decontamination without the concomitant use of protective isolation was investigated (Fig. 3c). The results are conflicting, although the same regimen was used for decontamination of the gut, i.e., a combination of gentamicin, vancomycin, and nystatin, given orally. Only Levine et al. (25) added topical antibiotics and antiseptics.

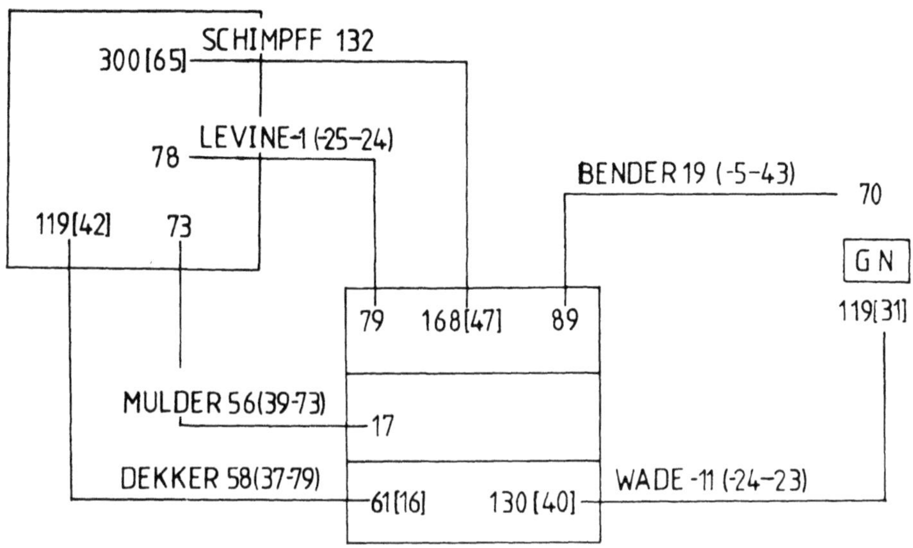

Fig. 3c. The effectiveness of total decontamination, partial decontamination and cotrimoxazole compared with standard care. See for legend Fig. 3b. GN = gentamicin and nystatin.

Schimpff et al. (26) reported a decrease in the number of infections in decontaminated patients, whereas Levine et al. (25) found no difference in the number of infections between control patients and decontaminated patients. This discrepancy is probably explained by the fact that Levine et al.'s control patients ran less risk of developing an infection than the decontamined patients did: the control patients spent twice as much of their time in the study with a granulocyte count higher than 1.0 x $10^9/1$ as the decontamined patients. The results of Schimpff et al. (26) were confirmed by a later publication giving the Baltimore group's experience with total decontamination in 87 granulocytopenic episodes of 70 patients (41). Bender et al. (42) (Fig. 3c) compared total decontamination with the combination of gentamicin, vancomycin, and nystatin with decontamination with gentamicin combined with nystatin, which does not give true total decontamination. There was no difference between the groups as to the infection rate, but colonization with Gram-negative aerobic micro-organisms was greater in the group treated with gentamicin, vancomycin, and nystatin.

Partial antibiotic decontamination

Only one study (43) has been published in which the effect of selective decontamination on the number of infections was compared with that in a control group, and no form of protective isolation was used (Fig. 3c). Selective decontamination was achieved by the oral administration of nalidixic acid, cotrimoxazole, or colistine, dosed according to the results of culture of the faeces and the pattern of resistance to antimicrobial agents in the cultured micro-organisms. Since use was made of cotrimoxazole in this study, the treatment cannot be called partial decontamination in the strict sense of this term. The number of infections in the selectively decontaminated patients was lower than that in the control group.

Cotrimoxazole

Hughes et al. (23), who studied the use of cotrimoxazole for the prevention of Pneumocystis carinii pneumonia, found a reduction not only in the number of infections with this micro-organism, but also in the number of bacterial infections. Fungal infections occurred more often in the cotrimoxazole-treated patients. These observations led to the use of cotrimoxazole in combination with an antifungal agent in the prevention of bacterial infections in granulocytopenic patients. Dekker et al. (44) studied the effect of cotrimoxazole combined with amphotericin B and nystatin on the number of infections in patients nursed in an open ward or single-bed room (Fig. 3c). Cotrimoxazole reduced the total number of infections relative to the number in control patients. This decrease was limited to infections of the skin, urinary tract, and soft tissues; there was no difference in the number of bacteremias and pulmonary infections. Wade et al. (45) compared the combination of gentamicin and nystatin with cotrimoxazole combined with nystatin and found them to be equally effective (Fig. 3c). Three studies (46-48) on trimethoprim alone compared with cotrimoxazole alone showed a higher number of trimethoprim-resistant micro-organisms in the patients on trimethoprim than in the patients on cotrimoxazole. The patients on cotrimoxazole also showed less colonization with potentially pathogenic micro-organisms. This means that trimethoprim alone is not a substitute for cotrimoxazole.

It may be concluded that antimicrobial decontamination without protective isolation reduces the infection rate. None of the methods of decontamination was found to be more effective than the others.

Effectiveness of the combination of protective isolation and decontamination

Many studies have been performed to investigate the effect of protective isolation combined with decontamination on the infection rate. For the present discussion, the methods of protective isolation applied have been divided into two groups: simple protective isolation (nursing in a single-bed room) and advanced protective isolation (nursing in a laminar airflow room or a plastic tent isolator). The regimens for decontamination investigated in the combination with simple protective isolation are fracon or neocon (neomycin, colistine, and nystatin)(49-51), cotrimoxazole alone (51-53) or with fracon (50,53), and partial antibiotic decontamination with the combination of polymyxine B, neomycin, amphotericin B and nalidixic acid (54,55)(Fig. 3d). Fracon combined with topical antiseptics and increasing of the drug dosages until enterobacteriaceae no longer appeared in the faeces cultures, reduced the number of infections relative to protective isolation alone (the infection rates being 52% and 98%, respectively), and was well tolerated by the patients (49). Comparison of the effectiveness of fracon with that of fracon plus cotrimoxazole showed fewer infections for the latter (infection rate 57%) than the former patients (infection rate 94%)(50). The difference in infection rate between the fracon-treated patients in the two studies is remarkable: 52% (49) and 94% (50), the latter equalling the infection rate in the control patients in the first study. This divergence was probably due to the abandonment of both the use of topical antiseptics and the adjustment of the dose of the antimicrobial drugs to achieve enterobacteriaceae-free faeces cultures, as inferred from the absence of any reference to these measures by the authors.

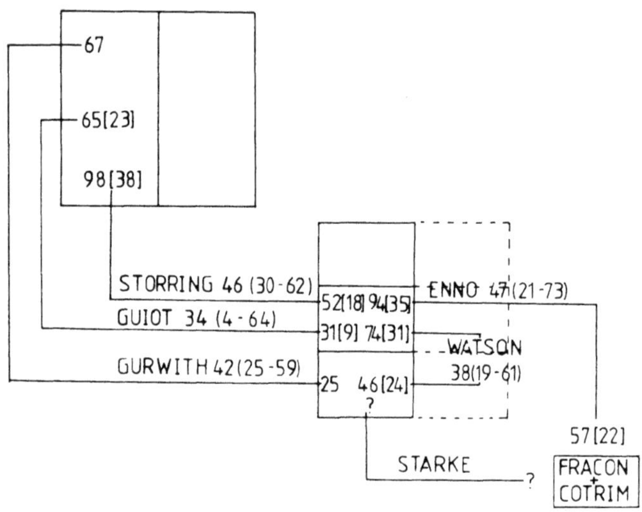

Fig. 3d. The effectiveness of decontamination and simple protective isolation compared with simple protective isolation alone. See for legend Fig. 3b.

Recently, the combination of fraco (fracon without nystatin) and cotrimoxazole was compared with cotrimoxazole alone in patients nursed in simple protective isolation (53). According to the authors, the two methods gave the same results, but cotrimoxazole is named as the drug of choice. However, when the faecal cultures of patients treated with cotrimoxazole showed cotrimoxazole-resistant micro-organisms, fraco was added or cotrimoxazole was changed to fraco. Of the 19 patients in the cotrimoxazole group, 5 acquired cotrimoxazole-resistant bacteria. How the patients that were switched to another regimen were evaluated is not described. The authors' conclusion cannot be verified and is doubtful: in fact, cotrimoxazole failed in 5 of the 19 patients.

In another recent study (51) the number of infections in patients treated with cotrimoxazole and nystatin or amphotericin B was lower (infection rate 46%) than that in patients treated with fracon (infection rate 74%). However, there was no difference in the number of bacteremias in the two groups, and of the 4 fatal cases in both groups, 1 patient in the fracon group and 3 in the cotrimoxazole group died of an infection. One patient was changed from cotrimoxazole to fracon because of a perianal abscess, and 10 patients had to stop taking cotrimoxazole because of adverse drug reactions. Gurwith (52) observed a reduction in the infection rate, especially of bacteremias and urinary-tract infections, when simple protective isolation was combined with the use of cotrimoxazole (infection rates 67% and 25%, respectively).

In a double blind placebo controlled clinical trial, we investigated (56) the effect of partial antibiotic decontamination (PAD) in patients with acute non-lymphocytic leukaemia nursed in simple protective isolation. The use of PAD reduced the number of infections, especially bacteremias involving aerobic Gram-negative bacteria (7 in the control group vs 1 in the PAD group). Two of the three major infections that occurred in patients on PAD were caused by micro-organisms that were not eliminated by PAD: one case of septicaemia caused by Streptococcus pneumoniae and one of a rectal infiltrate probably caused by anaerobic bacteria.

Total decontamination is the most extensively investigated regimen in combination with advanced protective isolation (25,26, 57-61)(Fig. 3c). The combination of antimicrobial drugs most often used for total decontamination is gentamicin, vancomycin, and nystatin (GVN)(25,26,57); variations are kanamycin, vancomycin, polymyxin B, and nystatin (60), paromomycin, vancomycin, polymycin B, and amphotericin B or nystatin (57); and bacitracin, neomycin, polymyxin B, and nystatin (59).

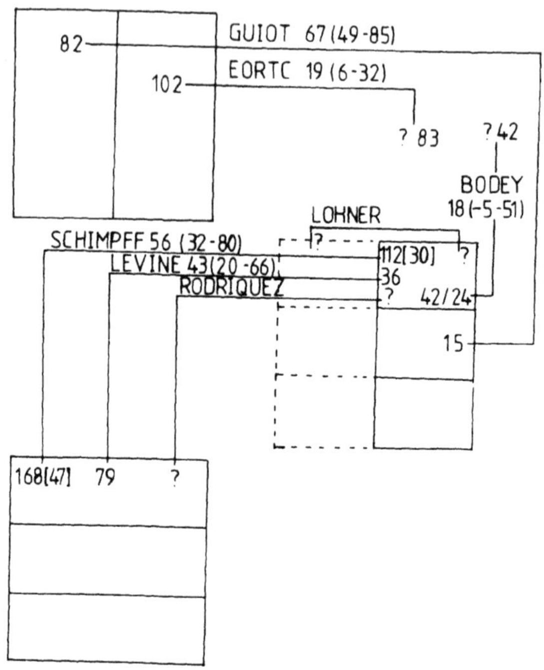

Fig. 3e. The effectiveness of decontamination and advanced protective isolation compared with one of those methods used alone. See for legend Fig. 3b.

Both Schimpff et al. (25) and Levine et al. (24) found a lower infection rate in patients decontaminated with GVN and nursed in protective isolation than in patients only decontaminated. Preisler (57) concluded from the results of a less than optimally designed investigation done in a small number of patients who were switched between groups and with the use of historical controls, that GVN with sterile food combined with nursing in laminar air flow rooms gave the highest number of negative faecal cultures, but this group also had the highest number of faecal cultures positive for fungi. The effect on the number of infections cannot be estimated from this report.

Bodey et al. (58) compared the infection rate in totally decontaminated patients nursed in protective isolation with that in historical controls whose treatment is not described. The infection rate was 24% for the decontaminated patients and 42% for the controls (mean of the two control groups). Some years later (28), the authors reported on the same regimen of decontamination and isolation in 102 episodes in 89 patients. Here, the frequency of major infections was 42%. Thus, it cannot be concluded from these data that decontamination and protective isolation in combination favoured the patients. The results of the decontamination, judged from the degree to which the patients became germ-free, are disappointing, since potentially pathogenic micro-organisms were present in 92 of the 102 episodes, which confirmed the earlier results of this kind of decontamination (27). These poor results have led to the use of a combination of orally non-absorbable and absorbable antibiotics and even to the use of systemically administered antibiotics (59). This systemic antibiotic prophylaxis did not give a better state of decontamination either, but the patients treated with this antibiotic prophylaxis in combination with protective isolation had fewer infections than the patients treated with the antibiotics alone.

The fact that it is very difficult, and perhaps impossible, to achieve a germ-free state by decontamination, was also shown by Dietrich et al. (61). A regimen of bacitracin, neomycin, polymyxin B, and nystatin resulted in sterile cultures of material from the skin, nose, and ears in about half of the patients, and 73% of the feacal cultures were sterile. In a multicentre trial (39) in which the method of decontamination was not standardized, the infection rates showed a small difference favouring the patients who had been decontaminated as well as isolated. Lohner et al. (60) reported a lower infection frequency in decontaminated patients nursed in laminar air flow rooms compared with patients nursed in single-bed rooms in a special-care ward and given sterile food.

With partial antibiotic decontamination in patients nursed in laminar air flow rooms the infection rate was 15% compared with 82% in the historical controls nursed in simple protective isolation (55). As already mentioned, this great reduction of the infection rate by partial antibiotic decontamination has been confirmed by a double blind placebo controlled clinical trial (56).

In sum, it may be said that the combination of protective isolation and antimicrobial decontamination reduces the infection rate more than either of the measures alone; and that antimicrobial decontamination with advanced protective isolation was not better than when combined with simple protective isolation.

Tolerability and patients' compliance

The regimens containing vancomycin are poorly tolerated, because of this drug's bad taste, although the patients' compliance was reported to be 80 to 85% (41,42), probably due to the continuing efforts to remind them of the great importance of taking the drugs. Cotrimoxazole is very well tolerated. In a comparative study the patients' compliance was better for cotrimoxazole and nystatin (94%) than for gentamicin and nystatin (73%)(45). In our trial on partial antimicrobial decontamination, the occurence of gastro-intestinal complaints was the same for the drug- and the placebo-treated patients (56). Complaints were associated with the cytostatic therapy more often than with the partial antimicrobial decontamination. Sterile food has a bad taste. Food with a low bacterial content is much more palatable and therefore better tolerated by the patients.

Unfavourable effects of antimicrobial decontamination

The main problem in total decontamination is colonization of the patient with multiresistant micro-organisms, including resistance to gentamicin, which is an important drug in the treatment of infections (41). The risk of colonization is greater in total decontamination than in partial decontamination or under cotrimoxazole therapy, because the latter two methods do not disturb the colonization resistance. Therefore, total decontamination seems to be safe only when it is combined with advanced protective isolation and the provision of sterile food. Although the risk of colonization is lower with cotrimoxazole than with total decontamination, the occurrence of micro-organisms resistant to sulfonamides and/or trimethoprim is a problem. Despite the initially optimistic view that resistance to cotrimoxazole would not occur (62-64), an ever-increasing number of reports mention the occurrence of resistance to this drug (44-47,53,65-68). The occurrence of resistant micro-organisms was also reported by Mulder et al. (43) to be a problem in the simple regimen for selective decontamination. No colonization with resistant micro-organisms has been seen with the broader regimen for partial decontamination we use (54-56).

The costs

Fig. 3f shows the costs per day for the various methods of protective isolation and antimicrobial decontamination. The fee for nursing in a Dutch university hospital in January, 1982, is taken as the cost of conventional care and protective isolation. The price of the drugs (shown between parentheses) for total decontamination was calculated for the combination of gentamicin, vancomycin, and nystatin, and those for partial antimicrobial decontamination as combined polymyxin B, neomycin, amphothericin B, and nystatin. The higher costs associated with these methods must be considered in relation to the gains afforded by lower numbers of infections and shorter hospitalization.

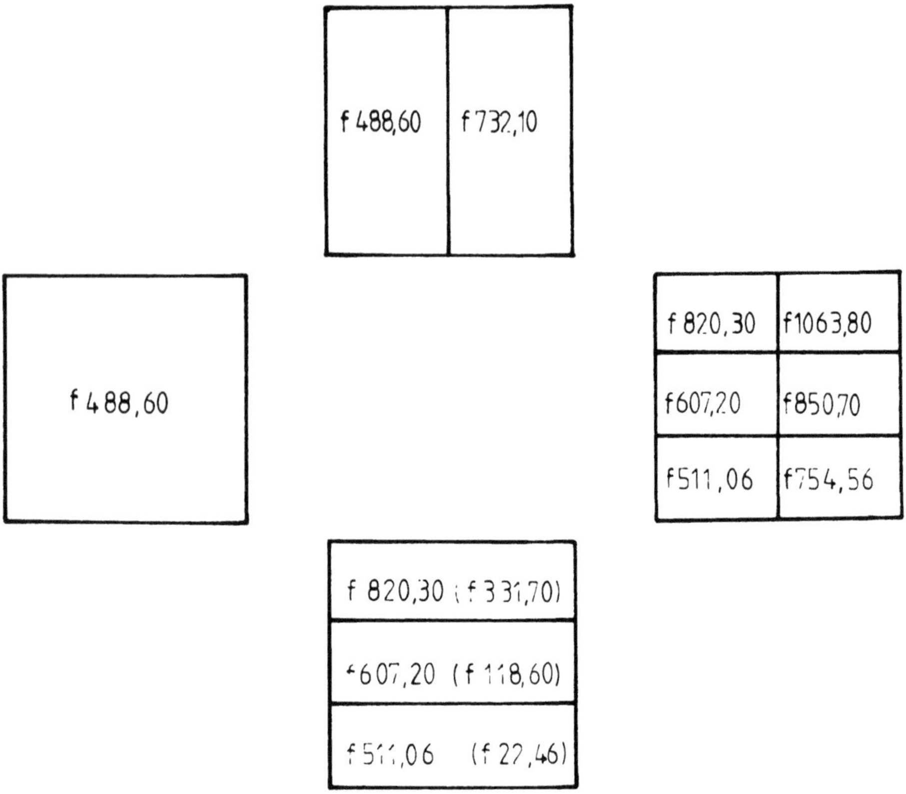

Fig. 3f. Costs per day of the various methods for protective isolation and antimicrobial decontamination (in Dutch guilders). Between parentheses: price of drugs alone.

CONCLUSIONS

With respect to effectiveness, none of the methods used for protective isolation or antimicrobial decontamination has proved to be superior to the others. A combination of protective isolation and antimicrobial decontamination is better than either of the methods alone. Total decontamination is badly tolerated, because of the vancomycin usually included in the regimen. Furthermore, because the risk of colonization is great due to the loss of colonization resistance, total decontamination must be combined with advanced protective isolation. Although cotrimoxazole does not influence colonization resistance, occurrence of cotrimoxazole-resistant micro-organisms is rather frequent. This disadvantage does not outweigh the low costs of this method. Partial antibiotic decontamination with simple protective isolation seems to be an effective, rather cheap, and safe method of prophylaxis for infections.

Table XI.

COMPARISON OF RESULTS OBTAINED WITH VARIOUS METHODS OF PROTECTIVE ISOLATION AND ANTIMICROBIAL DECONTAMINATION

	Efficacy	Tolerability	Untoward effects	Costs*
Simple isolation	good	good	no	±
Advanced isolation	good	moderate	no	++
Total decontamination	good	bad	yes	++
Partial decontamination	good	good	no	+
Cotrimoxazole	good	good	yes	±

* ++ = expensive; + = moderately expensive; ± = cheap

It must be kept in mind, however, that the prevention of hospital infections in immunocompromised patients must be based on measures taking into account the host defense, the patient's microbial flora and potential sources and chronic sites of infection, and specific prophylactic measures such as protective isolation and antimicrobial decontamination. To achieve effective prophylaxis of infection, attention must be paid to all of these measures; none may be neglected.

REFERENCES

1. Bodey, G.P. 1970. Epidemiological studies of Pseudomonas species in patients with leukaemia. Am. J. Med. Sci. 260: 82
2. Gurwith, M.J., Brunton, I.L., et al. 1978. Granulocytopenia in hospitalized patients. I. Prognostic factors and etiology of fever. Am. J. Med. 64: 121.
3. Schimpff, S.C., Moody, M., Young, V.M. 1970. Relationship of colonization with Pseudomonas aeruginsa to development of pseudomonas bacteremia in cancer patients. Antimicrob. Agents Chemother. 4: 240.
4. Schimpff, S.C., Young, V.M., et al. 1972. Origin of infection in acute non-lymphocytic leukaemia. Significance of hospital acquisition of potential pathogens. Ann. Intern. Med. 77: 707.
5. Levine, A.S., Schimpff, S.C., Graw, R.G., Young, R.C. 1974. Hematologic malignancies and other marrow failure states: Progress in the management of complicating infections. Semin. Hematol. 11: 141.
6. Nauta, E.H. 1979. Infection in the compromised host. In: G. Dick (ed.), Immunological aspects of infectious diseases. MTP Press Ltd., Lancaster.
7. Williams, D.M., Krick, J.A., Remington, J.S. 1976. Pulmonary infection in the compromised host. Am. Rev. Respir. Dis. 114: 359 (Part I) and 593 (Part II).
8. Meer van der, J.W.M., Broek van den, P.J. 1979. Infections in compromised patients. Diagnosic aspects. Neth. J. Med. 22: 108.
9. Valdivieso, M. 1976. Bacterial infection in haematological diseases. Clin. Haematol. 5: 229.
10. Bodey, G.P., Buckley, M., et al. 1966. Quantitative relationships between circulating leukocytes and infection i patients with acute leukaemia. Ann. Intern. Med. 64: 328.
11. Meer van der, J.W.M., Alleman, M., Boekhout, M. 1979. Infectious episodes in severely granulocytopenic patients. Infection 7: 171.
12. Hart, P.D., Russell, E., Remington, J.S. 1969. The compromised host and infection. II. Deep fungal infection. J. Inf. Dis. 120: 169.
13. Baker, R.D. 1962. Leukopenia and therapy in leukaemia as factors predisposing to fatal mycoses. Am. J. Clin. Pathol. 37: 358.
14. Colpin, G.G.D., Guiot, H.F.L., et al. 1981. Bacillus cerius meningitis in a patient under gnotobiotic care. Lancet ii: 694.
15. Price, D.J.E., Heigh, J.D. 1970. Control of infection due to Klebsiella aerogenes in a neurosurgical unit by withdrawal of all antibiotics. Lancet ii: 1213.
16. Greene, W.H., Schimpff, S.C., et al. 1973. Empiric carbenicillin gentamicin and cephalotin therapy for presumed infection in patients with granulocytopenia and cancer. Ann. Intern. Med. 78: 825.
17. Schimpff, S.C. 1977. Therapy of infection in patients with granulocytopenia. Med. Clin. North Am. 61: 1101.

18. Pollac, M., Charache, P. et al. 1972. Factors influencing colonization and antibiotic-resistance patterns of Gram-negative bacteria in hospital patients. Lancet ii: 668.
19. Pennington, J.E. 1977. Fever, neutropenia and malignancy: a clinical syndrome in evolution. Cancer 39: 1345.
20. Broek van der, P.J., Meer van der, J.W.M. 1979. Antimicrobial therapy in the myelo- and immunocompromised patient. Neth. J. Med. 22: 118.
21. Strauss, R.G., Connett, J.E., et al. 1981. A controlled trial of prophylactic granulocyte transfusions during initial induction chemotherapy for acute myelogenous leukaemia. N. Engl. J. Med. 305: 597.
22. Jones, R.J. 1981. Vaccines and antisera against Gram-negative bacilli. J. Hosp. Infect. 2: 105.
23. Hughes, W.T., Kuhn, S., et al. 1977. Successful chemoprophylaxis for Pneumocystis carinii pneumonitis. N. Engl. J. Med. 297: 1419.
24. McLaughlin, M.M., Dacquisito, M.P., et al. 1964. Effects of the germfree state on responses of mice to whole-body irradiation. Radiat. Res. 23: 333.
25. Levine, A.S. Siegel, S.E., et al. 1973. Protected environments and prophylactic antibiotics. A prospective controlled study of their utility in the therapy of acute leukaemia. N. Engl. J. Med. 288: 477.
26. Schimpff, S.C., Green, W.H., et al. 1975. Infection prevention in acute non-lymphocytic leukaemia. Laminar airflow room reverse isolation with oral, non-absorbable antibiotic prophylaxis. Ann. Intern. Med. 82: 351.
27. Bodey, G.P., Rosenbaum, B. 1974. Effect of prophylactic measures on the microbial flora of patients in protected environment units. Medicine 53: 209.
28. Bodey, G.P., Rodriques, V. 1975. Infections in cancer patients on a protected environment. Prophylactic antibiotic program. Am. J. Med. 59: 497.
29. Rodriquez, V., Bodey, G.P., et al. 1978. Randomized trial of protected environment. Prophylactic antibiotics in 145 adults with acute leukaemia. Medicine 57: 253.
30. Waay van der, D., Berghuis-de Vries, J.M., Lekkerkerk-Wees van der, J.E.C. 1971. Colonization resistance of the digestive tract in conventional and antibiotic-treated mice. J. Hyg. (Camb.) 69: 405.
31. Waay van der, D., Berghuis, J.M. 1974. Determination of the colonization resistance of the digestive tract of individual mice. J. Hyg. (Camb.) 72: 379.
32. Wulff, H.R. 1981. Rational diagnosis and treatment. Second edition. Blackwell Scientific Publications. Oxford, London, Edinburgh, Melbourne.
33. Lowbury, E.I.L., Babb, I.R., Ford, P.M. 1971. Protective isolation in a burns unit: The use of plastic isolators and air curtains. J. Hyg. (Camb.) 69: 529.
34. Cason, J.S., Jackson, D.M., et al. 1966. Antiseptic and aseptic prophylaxis for burns: Use of silver nitrate and of isolators. Br. Med. J. IV: 1288.
35. Lidwell, O.M., Towers, A.G. 1972. Unidirectional ("laminar") flow ventilation system for patient isolation. Lancet i: 347.

36. Winner, H.I., Bagshawe, K.D., et al. 1970. Microbiological aspects of cytotoxic drug therapy. Proc. R. Soc. Med. 63: 28.
37. Jameson, B., Gamble, R., et al. 1971. Five-year analysis of protective isolation. Lancet i: 1034.
38. Yates, J.W., Holland, J.F. 1973. A controlled study of isolation and endogenous microbial suppression in acute myelocytic leukaemia patients. Cancer 32: 1490.
39. Dietrich, M., Gaus, W., et al. 1977. Protective isolation and antimicrobial decontamination in patients with high susceptibility to infection. Infection 5: 107.
40. Nauseef, W.M., Maki, D.G. 1981. A study of the value of simple protective isolation in patients with granulocytopenia. N. Engl. J. Med. 304: 448.
41. Hahn, D.M., Schimpff, S.C., et al. 1978. Infection in acute leukaemia patients receiving oral non-absorbable antibiotics. Antimicrob. Agents Chemother. 13: 958.
42. Bender, J.F., Schimpff, S.C., et al. 1979. Role of vancomycin as a component of oral non-absorbable antibiotics for microbial suppression in leukaemic patients. Antimicrob. Agents Chemother. 15: 455.
43. Mulder, N.H., Nieweg, H.O., et al. 1979. Infection prevention in granulocytopenic patients by selective decontamination of the digestive tract. In: D. van der Waay and J. Verhoef (eds). New criteria for antimicrobial therapy. Excerpta Medica. Amsterdam, Oxford. 113.
44. Dekker, A.W., Rozenberg-Arska, M., et al. 1981. Prevention of infection by trimethoprim-sulfamethoxazole plus amphotericin B in patients with acute non-lymphocytic leukaemia. Ann. Intern. Med. 95: 555.
45. Wade, J.C., Schimpff, S.C., et al. 1981. A comparison of trimethoprim-sulfamethoxazole plus nystatin with gentamicin plus nystatin in the prevention of infections in acute leukaemia. N. Engl. J. Med. 304: 1057.
46. Gurwith, M.J., Trong, K. 1979. A comparison of prophylactic trimethoprim/sulfamethoxazole to trimethoprim alone in compromised hosts. Abstracts 11th ICC and 19th ICAAC, Boston, Massachusetts, U.S.A. Abstract 70.
47. McNaughton, R.D., Riben, P., et al. 1979. A comparison of trimethoprim and trimethoprim/sulfamethoxazole prophylaxis in neutropenic patients. The elimination of potential pathogens and the emergence of resistance. Abstracts 11th ICC and 19th ICAAC, Boston, Massachusetts, U.S.A. Abstract 69.
48. Guerrant, R.L., Wood, S.J., et al. 1981. Resistance among fecal flora of patients taking sulfamethoxazole-trimethoprim or trimethoprim alone. Antimicrob. Agents Chemother. 19:33.
49. Storring, R.A., Jameson, B., et al. 1977. Oral non-absorbed antibiotics prevent infection in acute non-lymphoblastic leukaemia. Lancet ii: 837.
50. Enno, A., Catovsky, D., et al. 1978. Cotrimoxazole for prevention of infection in acute leukaemia. lancet ii: 395.
51. Watson, J.G., Jameson, B., et al. 1982. Cotrimoxazole versu non-absorbable antibiotics in acute leukaemia. Lancet i: 6.

52. Gurwith, M.J., Brunton, J.C., et al. 1979. A prospective controlled investigation of prophylactic trimethoprim/ sulfamethoxazole in hospitalized granulocytopenic patients. Am. J. Med. 66: 248.
53. Starke, I.D., Donnelly, P., et al. 1982. Cotrimoxazole alone for prevention of bacterial infection in patients acute leukaemia. Lancet i: 5.
54. Guiot, H.F.L., Furth van, R. 1977. Partial antibiotic decontamination. Br. Med. J. I: 800.
55. Guiot, H.F.L., Meer van der, J.W.M., Furth van, R. 1981. Selective antimicrobial modulation of human microbial flora. Infection prevention in patients with decreased host defense mechanisms by selective elimination of potentially pathogenic bacteria. J. Infect. Dis. 143: 644.
56. Guiot, H.F.L., Broek van den, P.J., Meer van der, J.W.M., et al. 1982. Selective antimicrobial modulation of the intestinal flora as measure for infection prevention in patients with acute non-lymphocytic leukaemia. Submitted for publication.
57. Preisler, H.D., Goldstein, I.M., Henderson, E.S. 1970. Gastro-intestinal "sterilization" in the treatment of patients with acute leukaemia. Cancer 26: 1076.
58. Bodey, G.P., Gehan, E.A., et al. 1971. Protected environment-prophylactic antibiotic program in the chemotherapy of acute leukaemia. Am. J. Med. Sci. 262: 138.
59. Rodriquez, V., Bodey, G.P., et al. 1978. Randomized trial of protected environment-prophylactic antibiotics in 145 adults with acute leukaemia. Medicine 57: 253.
60. Lohner, D., Debusscher, L., et al. 1979. Comparitive randomized study of protected environment plus oral antibiotics versus oral antibiotics alone in neutropenic patients. Cancer Treat. Rep. 63: 363.
61. Dietrich, M., Rasche, H., et al. 1973. Antimicrobial therapy as a part of the decontamination procedures for patients with acute leukaemia. Eur. J. Cancer 9: 443.
62. Moorhouse, E.C., Farrell, W. 1972. Effect of cotrimoxazole on faecal enterobacteria. No emergence of resistant strains. J. Med. Microbiol. 6: 249.
63. Speller, D.C.E., Braten, D.M. 1972. Faecal flora after prolonged cotrimoxazole treatment. Br. Med. J. II: 416.
64. Knothe, H. 1973. The effect of a combined preparation of trimethoprim and sulphamethoxazole following short-term and long-term administration on the flora of the human gut. Chemotherapy 18: 285.
65. Mihara, G., Stamey, T.A. 1979. The effect of low-dose cotrimoxazole (trimethoprim-sulfamethoxazole) on rectal and vaginal flora. In: D. van der Waaij and J. Verhoef (eds). New criteria for antimicrobial therapy. Excerpta Medica. Amsterdam, Oxford. 243.
66. Murray, B.E., Rensimer, E.R., DuPont, H.L. 1982. Emergence of high-level trimethoprim resistance in fecal Escherichia coli during oral administration of trimethoprim or trimethoprim-sulfamethoxazole. N. Engl. J. Med. 306: 130.

67. Wilson, I.M., Guiney, D.G., 1982. Failure of oral trimethoprim-sulfamethoxazole prophylaxis in acute leukaemia. Isolation of resistant plasmids from strains of enterobacteriaceae causing bacteremia. N. Engl. J. Med. 306: 16.
68. Jacoby, G.A., 1982. Perils of prophylaxis (editorial). N. Engl. J. Med. 306: 43.

IMPLICATIONS AND CONSEQUENCES OF ANTIMICROBIAL THERAPY FOR THE DEVELOPMENT AND TRANSFER OF RESISTANCE

D. VAN DER WAAIJ

INTRODUCTION

Since antimicrobial drugs first became available for the treatment of infections, resistance has developed (1-12). The increase in the number of antibiotics and in the diversity of their spectrum of activity in the last few decades has not solved the problem: the use of new antibiotics has invariably led to the development of resistance after some time. Bacteria of many different species have proven to have an almost endless capacity to develop sublines of strains that are resistant, often to more than one antibiotic.

DEVELOPMENT OF RESISTANCE

The development of resistance rarely occurs at the site of the infection and can generally be prevented by adequate dosing of drugs possessing the right pharmacokinetic properties to reach the focus of the infection in an adequate concentration. As a rule, resistance to an antibiotic develops within the digestive tract. In the throat or in the intestinal lumen, resistance may develop among strains that are marginally susceptible to the (constantly varying) concentrations of the antibiotic. Virtually all anti-bacterial drugs are to some extent excreted with the saliva and/or the bile into the throat and intestinal lumen, respectively. Since the type of antibiotic selected for treatment, the dose, and the frequency of administration are determined by the species of bacteria isolated from the infection or -- if culture results are not available -- the bacteria thought to be involved in the infection, little attention is generally paid to what occurs in the alimentary canal during the treatment. The physician's only concern with respect to the patient's gastro-intestinal tract is the occurrence of side effects such as nausea and or diarrhoea, which give discomfort. However, the low and often varying concentration of the antibiotic prevailing in the oropharynx and/or intestines, favours the selection of resistant strains.

TRANSFER OF RESISTANCE

If the antibiotic is not only marginally suppressive for susceptible and potentially pathogenic strains, but is also suppressive for the anaerobic bacteria that play a role in colonization resistance (CR) (13,14), transfer of plasmids coding for antibiotic resistance may occur (15). At the same time, genetic information for adherence factors (16) -- whose transfer is questioned by some authors (17) -- or enterotoxin production may be exchanged in vivo (18). Transfer of plasmids by bacterial conjugation is possible in vivo when the CR is decreased, because a low CR permits a strong increase in the concentration of resistant strains (19). This is more generally known as bacterial overgrowth.

MUTATION AND SELECTION

During CR-decreasing antibiotic therapy, resistant and potentially pathogenic strains may proliferate to concentrations of as much as 10^9 bacteria per gram faeces. This number is about a thousand-fold higher than the average concentration of these bacteria when the CR is unaffected. Since bacteria may mutate once during each 10^6-10^8 divisions, the presence of (1000-fold) more bacteria implies a proportionally greater chance of the development of new mutants. Mutation and selection may concern not only resistance to an antibiotic but also adaptation of resistant bacteria permitting (easier) colonization of the oropharynx or the gut. Mutation may occasionally result in the development or modification of adherence-pili of bacteria such that the strain can better adhere to the mucosal lining. The fact that this event -- i.e., the change in a certain strain of a bacterial species making it capable of adherence to mucosal cells -- rarely occurs, could be explained by the fact that the majority of the mutations result in bacilli that are not compatible with survival in the alimentary canal. In this respect it is important to keep in mind that the time of treatment can be crucial. The longer a patient is treated with a CR-decreasing antibiotic which reaches only marignally effective concentrations in the intestinal lumen, the greater the chance that an undesirable (better colonizing) mutant will appear.

Development of resistance and of pili for mucosal adherence may occur less often when combinations of antibiotics are used for therapy, but since multi-resistant strains do occur, although they are relatively rare, mutation may even be possible under the conditions of multi-antibiotic therapy. Consequently, the use of combinations of antibiotics offers an improvement, but does not solve the problems of resistance and adherence.

CLINICAL CONSEQUENCES OF MUTATION AND SELECTION DURING ANTIBIOTIC TREATMENT

When we apply antibiotics clinically we should realize that the dramatic events outlined above may occur as they have apparently taken place since 1945 (1-12). In practice this means that when we select an antibiotic for therapy, we must not forget that we are about to treat not only an infection but also a patient with his or her microflora. The greater part of that predominantly anaerobic microflora contributes considerably to the CR of the patient's digestive tract, and is therefore highly beneficial to the patient. Maintenance of CR is particularly important during antibiotic therapy -- in an environment with a nosocomial flora, often consisting of (many) resistant strains -- because this mechanism controls the number of colonizing resistant potentially pathogenic micro-organisms, and thus can reduce the chance of a "superinfection".

ANTIMICROBIAL DRUGS AND COLONIZATION RESISTANCE

Experience in man (5,6,8,9,20-23) and screening tests in mice (24-27) have indicated that antimicrobial drugs can be classified according to their effect on CR. Some drugs are, like ampicillin and several other penicillins, strongly CR-suppressive. Other drugs exert no effect on CR, and a third group only has a negative influence on CR when given in relatively high daily doses. Antimicrobial drugs that are not CR-suppressive, are either almost completely absorbed in the small bowel after oral adminstration or undergo biliary excretion (oral cephalosporins), or else have a spectrum of activity that does not affect the anaerobic species participating in CR (e.g., polymixin, polyene antibiotics, co-trimoxazole, nalidixic acid, doxycyclin (28)). The intermediate group comprises mainly aminoglycosides and parenteral cephalosporins (26,28,29).

To avoid the development or transfer of resistance in vivo and to minimize the acquisition of (multi-)resistant strains during therapy, preference should be given to CR-indifferent drugs. However, resistance may still develop when only CR-indifferent drugs are used if no attention is paid to the amount of the drug that remains in the intestinal lumen after oral administration or is excreted into the digestive tract. If the dosage of such drugs is chosen solely to treat an infection, the fraction of the dose that remains or is excreted may be too low to suppress the potentially pathogenic flora in the intestinal canal (30). Experience to date has indicated that resistant strains may then emerge (1-12). To avoid the development of resistance or the transfer of plasmids in vivo, the dose of antibiotic for the treatment of an infection should either be so high that virtually all susceptible strains of potentially pathogenic bacteria which colonize the alimentary tract are fully suppressed, or else so low that concentrations occur which are well below the minimal inhibitory concentration of the colonizing potentially pathogenic micro-organisms.

When CR-decreasing antibiotics are indicated for the treatment of an infection -- for example, because the bacterium involved in the infection is resistant to CR-indifferent drugs, or because the patient is allergic to proper CR-indifferent drugs -- a treatment combining systemic CR-decreasing antibiotics with non-absorbable CR-indifferent drugs should be considered. Overgrowth of the digestive tract by resistant bacteria or yeasts during CR-decreasing therapy can as a rule be limited effectively or even prevented, if the patient is concomitantly treated orally with a polyene antibiotic (amphotericin B or nystatin) to control yeast proliferation and polymyxin B or E for the supression of (most) Gram-negative bacilli. Obviously, these CR-indifferent oral drugs must be used in sufficiently high and frequent doses to produce within the alimentary tract a cidal concentration for Candida species and susceptible Gram-negative bacilli, respectively. For example, in adult patients amphotericin B should be given in four daily doses of 0.5 g and polymyxin in four daily doses of 200 mg each (30). If the patient who is systemically treated with CR-decreasing antibiotics is colonized by Proteus species -- which are naturally resistant to polymyxin -- or when nosocomial polymyxin-resistant strains are present in the ward, the use of low oral doses of 80 mg tobramycin four times a day, in addition to oral polymyxin, is in most cases adequate to control overgrowth by polymyxin-resistant Gram-negative bacilli (24). Gram-positive bacteria, such as Staphylococcus aureus, that are resistant to the CR-decreasing drug selected for therapy, may soon disappear from the oropharynx after treatment with cephradine in four daily doses of 1.5 g (30).

SELECTIVE DECONTAMINATION OF THE DIGESTIVE TRACT

The application of (oral) CR-indifferent drugs in doses that are suppressive to the patient's potentially pathogenic flora has become known in recent years as selective decontamination (SD). When the drugs in question are properly dosed and the combination applied is adjusted to the patient's admission flora as well as to the nosocomial flora in the ward, SD has been proven to be an important method for infection prophylaxis in severely neutropenic patients (31,33-37). Insufficient dosing of CR-indifferent drugs for SD (38) and the combination of CR-indifferent with CR-decreasing drugs for infection prophylaxis (39), have proved to be less successful.

SUMMARY

The use of antimicrobial drugs without taking into consideration their effect on the digestive-tract microflora, can lead to resistance, overgrowth, and superinfections. According to their effect on the alimentary-tract flora, anti-microbial drugs can be divided into two groups: 1. drugs which suppress the (anaerobic) flora determining colonization resistance, and 2. antimicrobial agents which leave the flora responsible for colonization resistance unchanged. The first category of antibiotics will not cause overgrowth by resistant micro-organisms. They can even be successfully applied for infection prophylaxis in neutropenic patients, provided the dosage is sufficiently high to completely suppress all susceptible potentially pathogenic microbes colonizing the digestive tract. This application of CR-indifferent drugs is called selective decontamination (SD). Antibiotics which decrease CR by suppressing CR-promoting (anaerobic) bacteria in the alimentary canal, should be considered second-choice antibiotics, particularly in a clinical setting. If use of the latter drugs is indicated by the sensitivity pattern of the micro-organisms involved in an infection, by their pharmacokinetic properties, or by the patient's kidney function or an allergy for CR-indifferent drugs, a combination of SD and therapy with such drugs should be considered.

REFERENCES

1. Julianelle, L.A., Siegel, M. 1945. The epidemiology of acute respiratory infections conditioned by sulfonamides. II. Gross alterations in the naso-pharyngeal flora associated with treatment. Ann. Int. Med. 22: 10.
2. Weinstein, L. 1947. The spontaneous occurrence of new bacterial infections during the course of treatment with streptomycin or penicillin. Am. J. Med. 214: 56.

3. Smith, D.T. 1952. The disturbance of the normal bacterial ecology by the administration of antibiotics with the development of new clinical syndromes. Ann. Int. Med. 27: 1135.
4. Louria, D.B., Kaminski, Th. 1962. The effects of four antimicrobial drug regimens on sputum superinfection in hospitalized patients. Am. Rev. Resp. Dis. 85: 649.
5. Finegold, S.M., Harada, N.E., Miller, L.G. 1965. Lyncomycin: Activity against anaerobes and effect on normal human fecal flora. Antimicrob. Agents Chemother. 5: 659.
6. Sompolinski, D., Yaron, V., Alkan, W.J. 1967. Microbiological changes in the human fecal flora following the administration of tetracyclines and chloramphenicol. Am. J. Proctol. 18: 471.
7. Rose, H.D., Schreier, J. 1968. The effect of hospitalization and antibiotic therapy on the Gram-negative fecal flora. Am. J. Med. Sci. 255: 228.
8. Shaw, E.J., Datta, N., Jones, G., Marr, F.M., Froud, W.K.B. 1973. Effect of stay in hospital and oral chemotherapy on the antibiotic sensitivity of bowel coliforms. J. Hyg. 71: 529.
9. Hirsh, D.C., Burton, G.C., Blenden, D.C. 1974. The effect of tetracycline upon establishment of Escherichia coli of bovine origin in the enteric tract of man. J. Appl. Bact. 37: 327.
10. Gaman, W., Cates, C., Snelling, C.F.T., Lank, B., Ronald, A.R. 1976. Emergence of gentamicin- and carbicillin-resistant Pseudomonas aeruginosa in a hospital environment. Antimicrob. Agents Chemother. 9: 474.
11. Roberts, N., Douglas, R.G. 1978. Gentamicin use and Pseudomonas and Serratia resistance: Effect of a surgical prophylaxis regimen. Antimicrob. Agents Chemother. 13: 214.
12. Chow, A.W., Taylor, Ph.R., Yoshikawa, T.T., Guze, L.B. 1978. A nosocomial outbreak of infections due to multiply resistant Proteus mirabilis: Role of intestinal colonization as a major reservoir. J. Inf. Dis. 139: 621.
13. Waaij van der, D., Vries de, J.M., Lekkerkerk, J.E.C. 1971. Colonization resistance of the digestive tract in conventional and antibiotic-treated mice. J. Hyg. 69:405.
14. Waaij van der, D. 1979. The colonization resistance of the digestive tract in man and animals. Zbl. Bakt. Suppl. 7: 155.
15. Laufs, R., Fock, R., Von Hülst, F.B., Ritter, R. 1979. Transfer of R-factors during antibiotic treatment in the hospital. In: New Criteria for antimicrobial therapy: Maintenance of digestive tract colonization resistance. Eds D. van der Waaij, J. Verhoef. Excerpta Medica. Amsterdam, Oxford. 74.
16. Evans, D.G., Silver, R.P., Evans, D.J., Chase, D.G., Gorbach, S.L. 1975. Plasmid-controlled colonization factor associated with virulence in Escherichia coli enterotoxin for humans. Infect. Immun. 12: 656.
17. Nandadasa, H.G., Sargent, G.F., Brown, M.G.M., McNeish, A.S., Williams, P.H. 1981. The role of plasmids in adherence of adhesive Escherichia coli to mammalian cells. J. Inf. Dis. 143: 286.

18. Echeverria, P., Murphy, J.R. 1980. Enteroxigenic Escherichia coli carrying plasmids coding for antibiotic resistance and enterotoxin production. J. Inf. Dis. 142: 273.
19. Waaij van der, D. 1979. Th colonization resistance of the digestive tract in experimental animals and its consequence for infection prevention, acquisition of new bacteria and the prevention of spread of bacteria between cage mates. In: New criteria for antimicrobial therapy: Maintenance of digestive tract colonization resistance. Eds D. van der Waaij, J. Verhoef. Excerpta Medica. Amsterdam, Oxford. 43.
20. Louria, D.B., Brayton, R.G : 1963. The efficacy of penicillin regimens: With observations on the frequency of superinfections. JAMA 186: 987.
21. Gorbach, S.L., Spanknebel, G., Weinstein, L., Plant, A.G., Nahas, L., Levitan, R. 1969. Studies of intestinal microflora. VIII. Effect of Lincomycin on the microbial population of the human intestine. J. Inf. Dis. 120: 298.
22. Hinton, N.A. 1970. The effect of oral tetracyclin-HCl and doxycycline on the intestinal flora. Curr. Ther. Res. 12: 341.
23. Hartley, Ch.L, Clements, H.M., Linton, K.B. 1977. Effects of cephalexin erythromycin and clindamycin on the anerobic Gram-negative faecal flora in man. J. Med. Microbiol. 11: 125.
24. Thijm, H.A., Waaij van der, D. 1979. The effect of three frequently applied antibiotics on the colonization resistance of the digestive tract of mice. J. Hyg. 82: 397.
25. Emmelot, C.H., Waaij van der, D. 1980. The dose at which neomycin and polymixin B can be applied for selective decontamination of the digestive tract in mice. J. Hyg. 84: 331.
26. Waaij van der, D., Aberson, J., Thijm, A.H., Welling, G.W. 1982. The screening of four aminoglycosides in the selective decontamination of the digestive tract in mice. Infection 10: 35.
27. Wiegersma, N., Jansen, G., Waaij van der, D. 1982. Effect of twelve antimicrobial drugs on the colonization resistance of the digestive tract of mice an on endogenous potentially pathogenic bacteria. J. Hyg. In press.
28. Waaij van der, D. 1979. Colonization resistance of the digestive tract as a major lead in the selection of antibiotics for therapy. In: New criteria for antimicrobial therapy: Maintenance of digestive tract colonization resistance. Eds D. van der Waaij, J. Verhoef. Excerpta Medica. Amsterdam, Oxford. 271.
29. Waaij van der, D., Hofstra, W., Wiegersma, N. 1982. The effect of two cephalosporins and two broad-spectrum penicillins on the colonization resistance of the digestive tract. J. Inf. Dis. In press.
30. Murray, B.E., Rensimer, E.D., DuPont, H.L. 1982. Emergence of high-level trimethoprim resistance in fecal Escherichia coli during oral administration of trimethoprim or trimethoprim-sulfamethoxazole. N. Engl. J. Med. 306: 130.

31. Sleijfer, D.Th., Mulder, N.H., Vries de-Hospers, H.G., Fidler, V., Nieweg, H.O., Waaij van der, D., Saene van, H.K.F. 1980. Infection prevention in granulocytopenic patients by selective decontamination of the digestive tract. Eur. J. Cancer 16: 859.
32. Saene van, H.K.F., Driessen, L.H.M.N. 1979. Importance of the treatment of Staphylococcus aureus carriership in the prevention and therapy of Staphylococcus aureus infections. In: New criteria for antimicrobial therapy: Maintenance of digestive tract colonization resistance. Eds D. van der Waaij, J. Verhoef. Excerpta Medica. Amsterdam, Oxford. 197.
33. Vries de-Hospers, H.G., Sleijfer, D.Th., Mulder, N.H., Waaij van der, D., Nieweg, H.O., Saene van, H.K.F. 1981. Bacterial aspects of selective decontamination of the digestive tract as a method of infection prevention in granulopenic patients. Antimicrob. Agents Chemother. 19: 813.
34. Guiot, H.F.L., Meer van der, J.W.M., Furth van, R. 1981. Selective antimicrobial modulation of human microbial flora. Infection prevention in patients with decreased host defense mechanisms by selective elimination of potentially pathogenic bacteria. J. Inf. Dis. 143: 644.
35. Jehn, U., Ruckdeschell, G., Saner, H., Clemm, Ch., Wilmans, W. 1981. Vergleichende Studie zum Wert der Selektiven Darmdekontamination (SDD) bei der Behandlung akuter leukämien. Klin. Wochenschr. 59: 1093.
36. Kurrle, E. 1981. Infektprophylaxe bei der Induktion Therapie akuter leukämien. Klin. Wochenschr. 59: 1085.
37. Dekker, A.W., Rozenberg-Arska, M., Sixma, J.J., Verhoef, J. 1982. Prevention of infection by co-trimoxazole in patients with acute non-lymphocytic leukemia. Ann. Int. Med. 95: 555.
38. Wilson, J.M., Guiney, D.G. 1982. Failure of oral trimethoprim-sulfamethoxazole prophylaxis in acute leukaemia. N. Engl. J. Med. 306: 16.
39. Watson, J.G., Powels, R.L., Lawson, D.N., Morgenstern, G.R., Jameson, B., McElwain, T.J., Judson, I., Lumley, H., Kay, H.E.M. 1982. Co-trimoxazole versus non-absorbable antibiotics in acute leukaemia. Lancet i: 6.

DISCUSSION EDITED BY D. VAN DER WAAIJ*

The subjects discussed were: similarities and differences between partial antiboitc decontamination (PAD) and selective decontamination (SD); co-trimoxazole as single drug in infection prophylaxis; interval between the onset of treatment and the first negative cultures in decontamination; necessity for isolation of patients during PAD or SD; necessity for reconventionalization by oral feeding of anaerobes after beta-lactam antibiotic therapy during PAD or SD; availability of life tables and other parameters in cost-benefit calculation; and application of SD in other patient categories.

Partial antibiotic decontamination (PAD) and selective decontamination (SD) both aim at the reduction of potentially pathogenic micro-organisms qualitatively as well as quantitatively. During such treatment, the anaerobic flora is spared in order to keep the colonization resistance (CR) of the digestive tract as high as possible. In PAD a standard regimen of antimicrobial drugs is used, whereas in SD the treatment is started with a modifiable combination, for example co-trimoxazole and colistin together with a polyene antibiotic. Thrice-weekly monitoring of the patient's flora permits rapid readjustment of the combination when necessary; i.e., if a bacterium resistant to one or more of the drugs used for decontamination is found to be present, the treatment regimen is changed in accordance with the sensitivity pattern of the strain(s) isolated.

* Participants in the discussion: van den Broek, van Furth, Guiot, Hoogkamp, van der Meer, Nauta, Rubin, Thompson, Young, van der Waaij.

The interval between the start of treatment and the first negative cultures depends on the drug(s) used: for co-trimoxazole and nalidix acid, when given alone, this period is 5-7 days, whereas non-absorbable antibiotics such as polymyxin (colinstin) and (low-dose) neomycin have a more rapid effect. This divergence might be explained by the finding in animals that the first two drugs act mainly at the mucosal site, since they appear to be excreted with the mucus, whereas both of the non-absorbable antibiotics become mixed with the intestinal contents. Mucus containing co-trimoxazole or nalidixic acid prevents adherence of susceptible bacteria; peristaltic movement ultimately eliminates the non-adhering flora in about a week. Co-trimoxazole has been used in Utrecht as a single drug for infection prophylaxis: as in other centres, the results were relatively disappointing, and the drug was found to be inferior to the PAD regimen. Furthermore, evidence has been obtained that co-trimoxazole may interfere with bone marrow repopulation after chemotherapy.

Protective isolation may enhance the effect of PAD, although it was felt that the main attention should be given to the microbiological status of food and beverages, which should have a low contamination level. In SD so far (more than 200 patients), no special measures have been applied except normal hygienic hospital conditions, since the flexibility of the treatment regime permits quick response to colonization by resistant strains. Oral contamination with high numbers of resistant bacteria must, however, be prevented at any price, also in SD patients, because this exposure can lead rapidly to infection.

Reconventionalization is occasionally performed in Leiden in patients whose anaerobic flora is found to have been severely reduced by beta-lactam antibiotic therapy instituted for the treatment of a systemic infection. For this purpose, faeces (anaerobic flora) of a successfully PAD-treated patient are washed several times and then given orally in chocolate milk to the deficient patient. This generally leads to rapid recolonization of the colon with anaerobic bacteria.

Patients given SD were rarely treated systemically with a beta-lactam antibiotic when an infection was suspected on clinical grounds. Instead, CR-indifferent antibiotics such as the combination of cefradine and tobramycin, were given i.v. This treatment does not harm the anaerobic flora.

Life tables are not available for PAD- or SD-treated patients. The diversity of the diagnoses and thus of immunosuppressive treatment was put forward to explain why no reliable information is available yet on this point. It was doubted whether PAD or SD would add substantially to the ultimate life-span of patients with acute leukaemia. The low incidence of severe infections (which reduces the need for not only granulocyte transfusions but also expensive antibiotics), the improved quality of life for the patients on a decontamination regimen during phases with severe granulocytopenia, and the low grade of isolation required, all reduce the costs of treatment considerably. Although the life of leukaemia patients is ultimately not prolonged by this kind of antimicrobial prophylaxis, which is only a supportive treatment, it improves the quality of their life. Finally, the mortality due to infections in decontaminated patients was lower in both PAD- and SD-treated patients.

The applicability of SD to other patient categories is being investigated in the University Hospital Groningen. The high-risk patients in the intensive care unit of the Department of Surgery -- patients who are intubated for a week or longer, often while unconscious and often with an infection at admission -- are treated with SD. In such patients, special attention is paid to SD of the oropharynx. This approach has not only proved very benificial to the patients thus treated but also appeared to have considerable implications for the epidemiology in that ward. Before the SD regimen was instituted, the high-risk category of patients formed -- despite the usual measures taken to prevent transfer of such bacteria from patient to patient -- an important reservoir of mainly multi-resistant (Gram-negative) bacteria.

DON'T TOUCH THE BLADE: CONTROL OF SURGICAL SEPSIS

O.M. LIDWELL

INTRODUCTION

I take my title from an account of a veterinary operation in a remote mining community in mid-Norway in the 17th century. "He passed the knives and forceps over the fire, moving them always with the sun. By fire he might render the evil harmless. As he did so he murmured a spell. The instruments were so easily bewitched when they cut into living flesh. When all were prepared he wrapped them in a newly washed linen cloth, bleached by moonlight and handed the bundle to his assistant. Give them to me in order, but pass them with the sun and DONT TOUCH THE BLADE".(1). This, with its description of "rational" preparations, carried out with little or no understanding of their significance, mixed with ritual manoeuvres "sanctified by use without any test of their effectiveness" (2), might have been written as a parody of present day operating room practice. Without an understanding of the way in which infection and sepsis arise in surgical wounds it is impossible to devise effective methods of control and to eliminate inherited procedures which, even if harmless in themselves, absorb hard won time and effort. It is a difficult decision to discontinue time-honoured practices, or even recent innovations supported by an opinion that this must be benficial.

Surely we can omit the bleaching by moonlight, it is very inconvenient and time consuming and the nurses object ; after all, there is no evidence that it does any good. But listen : "... it would be a rather imprecise scientific experiment to simplify some procedures and wait to see whether ... infection developed ... such experiments are probably not ethical since

... patients might be harmed"(3). If we do omit it and an infection follows, as it will, the patient or his representatives may sue ; better be on the safe side.

The decision is not made any easier by the impossibility of ever proving conclusively that any practice is totally ineffective. As table 1 shows the number of observations required to demonstrate, in a controlled trial, that any specific measure has an effect on the incidence of sepsis increases without limit the smaller the proportionate effect.

Table 1.
NUMBER OF OBSERVATIONS REQUIRED

Infection rate without measure	10 %	5 %	2 %	1 %
Percentage reduction due to measure				
100	180	380	1.0×10^3	2.0×10^3
50	1.1×10^3	2.3×10^3	5.9×10^3	1.2×10^4
20	8.5×10^3	1.8×10^4	4.5×10^4	9.0×10^4
10	3.6×10^4	7.4×10^4	1.9×10^5	3.8×10^5

The numbers given relate to the total numbers of observations, control and treated together, with equal numbers in the two groups. Situations above and to the left of the broken line can be evaluated with fewer than 1000 observations. Those below and to the right of the full line need more than 10.000.

Most detailed procedures must, therefore, be determined by deduction from general principles ; although they may also, sometimes, as we shall see later, be supported by bacteriological evidence.

THE GERM THEORY OF DISEASE

So we need a unifying theory to serve as a working hypothesis. This was first provided by Listers' interpretation of Pasteurs' observations (4). His line of thought was this. Surgical sepsis is analogous to putrefaction, due to the multiplication of micro-organisms in the exposed tissue. For this to occur there must be : 1. a source of micro-organisms ; 2. they must be transferred into the wound ; 3. they must multiply there. If we can eliminate any of these three steps then sepsis cannot arise. Lister had little information on the first, except that micro-organisms were widely distributed. He chose phenol as an agent, in the first place to inhibit the third step, but later in an attempt to prevent the second, both via the air, with the famous spray and from any object which was brought into contact with the wound.

The success of these measures not only confirmed the usefulness of the hypothesis but also provided a starting point from which more detailed understanding could be gained.

SOURCES OF MICRO-ORGANISMS IN THE OPERATING ROOM

All surgery exposes potentially susceptible tissue to the possibility of infection. The scalpel itself and the other instruments and materials used may carry infection. The surgeons hands can only be clean, never sterile, nor can the patients skin. Each person in the operating room carries a rich variety of micro-organisms, many of which are plentifully and continuously shed on skin squames, small enough to pass through the pores of most woven materials and to be dispersed into the air and carried on every current. Bacterially contaminated air may also enter the operating room from other parts of the suite or the hospital. If internal viscera are punctured in the course of the surgical proceedings a heavy load of bacteria may be discharged into the wound.

The sources are many but it is the human sources that are the most intractable. Properly controlled sterilisation procedures will ensure that no contamination reaches the wound from instruments or materials so long as these are not contaminated from the operating room environment - don't touch the blade, once it has been cleansed. All micro-organisms are equal - there is no sharp dividing line between the pathogenic and the others. Given suitable conditions practically speaking any species may produce sepsis - but some are more equal than others.

In spite of premature announcements of its demise as a major source of wound sepsis, staphylococcus aureus is still among the front runners. Since carriage by operating room staff is detectable it would seem a rational step to discover and exclude these sources. The frequency of carriage is such that this apparently simple procedure is not really practicable. However, if an outbreak of infection with a particular strain occurs, the carrier(s) of the strain should be sought out and treated. This demands vigilance and regular phage-typing of wound strains. No one with a boil, an infected skin lesion or colonized eczema should work in the operating room. Infections with streptococcus pyogenes are also dangerous and respiratory infections expose the patient to risk at a time when he or she may be particularly susceptible. The patient himself is also a source of potential infection and the above considerations apply equally but may have to be overidden if operation cannot be delayed. The importance of different species of micro-organisms in relation to surgical infection is illustrated in tables 2 and 3.

Table 2.
AUTOGENOUS WOUND INFECTION WITH STAPHYLOCOCCUS AUREUS

	Infections/1000 patients	
	Infected with own strain	Infected with extraneous strain
Carrier of Staphylococcus aureus	27	18
Non-carrier	-	13

After Bengtsson et al (15).

Table 3.
BACTERIAL SPECIES FOUND IN INFECTED WOUNDS

	Operation type		
	Contaminated	Clean	Joint-replacement
Number of wounds	98	102	86
Species found			
Staphylococcus aureus	32	44	27
Streptococcus pyogenes	4	4	-
Staphylococcus albus	5	15	16
Propionibacterium	-	-	6
Other skin commensals	-	-	6
Above as percentage of all species	43	67	81
Gram-negative bacilli	62	22	11
Enterococci	8	4	4
Anaerobes	13	8	1
Above as percentage of all species	87	36	24
None isolated	3	8	18

Compiled from Bengtsson et al (15) and the multi-hospital investigation (12).

The large part played by endogenous sources in infection of "contaminated" wounds, which include those where the gut was entered, is apparent, as is also the role of patient staphylococcal carriage. The joint replacement operations illustrate not only a predominance of organisms probably originating from the skin but also the relatively large contribution, in this sensitive situation, of organisms often discounted as insignificant on grounds of negligible pathogenicity. It is only in recent years that greater attention to sampling and cultural mehtods has demonstrated that many "sterile" infections were due to these species, including the anaerobic skin flora. These technical improvements have also revealed the importance of other previously unrecognized anaerobic species e.g. bacteroides spp. as endogenous sources of infection.

TRANSFER INTO THE WOUND

Lister originally thought the evil was in the air and initiated his antiseptic method on this assumption. However he did not ignore other possibilities and disinfected sutures and swabs, treating also his own hands and the patients skin. In the end he became convinced that the numbers of organisms which might reach the wound from the air were too few to initiate sepsis. ".... (if) we can trust ourselves and our assistants to avoid the introduction into the wound of septic defilement ...." (5). Contact, touch, seemed to be the all important consideration. In this conclusion, at that time, he was surely more than 90 % right.

The surgeons hands come into the most intimate contact with the wound. The long tradition of the extended pre-operative scrub with soap and water followed by the donning of sterile rubber gloves received then a double shock with the revelation that this treatment was almost entirely ineffective in removing the resident skin flora of the handsand that a very high proportion of gloves exhibited punctures when examined after the end of the operation. This is a good example of an area where laboratory and bacteriological studies have combined to question existing practice and to provide a rational improvement where clinical evaluation is probably impracticable. Soil and extraneous micro-organisms can be removed by simple washing ; and the use of alcohol, alone or combined with disinfectants, gives a very large reduction in the numbers of the skin flora, which persists or improves over several hours within the gloved hand. Under these conditions emergence of bacteria through holes in the gloves is almost completely eliminated (6, 7).

But, is touch all ? The instruments are so easily bewitched ; if they cut into living flesh. Micro-organisms of species capable of and known to cause surgical sepsis are present in the air of every operating room, some must settle into the wound and onto instruments and material exposed within the room. The problem is a quantitative as well as a qualitative one.

If asepsis is poor contact will introduce into the wound numbers of micro-organisms far in excess of any which can arrive directly from the air. Air contamination is then irrelevant and we waste our money by playing with expensive schemes for special ventilation. The same applies to "contaminated" wounds.

If, however, we are concerned with clean surgery and asepsis is good then, perhaps, a rather high level of air contamination may be the dominant contributor to wound infection. In this case the introduction of a "good" ventilation system and attention to those activities which lead to excessive airborne dispersal may be advantageous.

The qualitative aspect arises from the differing susceptability of operated sites to infection. In particular the introduction of a foreign body e.g. some form of prosthesis, provides a site which can be colonized by organisms of negligible pathogenicity to normal tissue. It also may derive from the particular source from which an infecting organism can be transferred, e.g. clostrida are a normal part of the gut flora and clostridial infection of high-level leg-amputation arises normally from this, autogenous, source (9).

The relevance of air-borne infection to surgery has been for more than a century one of the most controversial points in surgery. Following Lister's final scepticism medical opinion generally dismissed it. But sepsis remained and with the returning swing of the pendulum renewed attention was directed towards the air as a possible vehicle for the bacterial innoculation of wounds. The idea was pursued with considerable vigour in the post war years of the fifties. Many studies of ventilation systems then demonstrated that reduced levels of airborne contamination resulted from these ; and led to a widely accepted specification for acceptable standards of operating room ventilation (8), i.e. a filtered air supply of at least 0.5 m^3/sec., arranged so as to produce a small positive air pressure between the operating room and its immediate surrounding, thereby both removing air-borne particles dispersed into the room and excluding contaminated air from outside. However, although there were many reports of improvements in the incidence of surgical sepsis after the introduction of such improved ventilation there were no controlled studies to confirm that the improvement was a consequences of the reduction in air-borne contamination (10).

A further impetus was given to the consideration of ultra-clean - air systems i.e. those leading to air - contamination levels at least 10 times lower than those resulting from the "standard" specification given above, by the enormous development over the following decades of implant surgery particularly the insertion of the artificial hip-joint. These operations, brilliant examples of reparative surgery, laid open to infection in thousands tissue highly susceptible to infection in the presence of a foreign body ; and infection followed. Sir John Charnley who had been one of the foremost pioneers in the surgical development now vigorously pursued the ideal of an aseptic operating environment by employing ultraclean air techniques (11). As was the case with Lister a century earlier, a steady reduction in the incidence of sepsis, from around 10 % to below 1 %, followed. But again, repeating the earlier situation, may other changes in technique accompanied the provision of cleaner air and a convincing causal relationships was not established.

INNOCULATION, INFECTION, SEPSIS

From the previous discussion it must appear that few surgical wounds can escape the introduction of bacterial contamination. Only a minority, however, develop disease. Is this a chance event or could it be predicted and hence, perhaps, prevented ? Manifestly some sites are more prone to infection than others, the beneficial effect of a good blood supply has long been recognized. Conversely we have already referred to the influence of a foreign body in facilitating bacterial growth. Clot or necrotic tissue left in the wound will similarly assist the development of infection. Some bacterial species are more invasive than others, and this ability is related to the body site involved and its condition. The wet treatment of burns encourages pseudomonas, exposure and dryness is more favourable to streptococcal infection. Clostridia will only multiply in an oxygen deficient environment. Less understood are the effects of host factors, both differences between patients and in the state of the same patient at different times. This is an important area for future study. Akin to the antagonistic action of host factors in the presence of intruding micro-organisms is that of systemic antibiotics. There is a critical distinction here between their prophylactic use and use for the treatment of an established infection. In the later case it should be possible to assess the susceptability of the infecting organism and institute a suitable antibiotic regime. In the first case it becomes a question of predicting the most probable infecting organism or organisms. There are some clear cut situations. Thus gas gangrene following high-level amputation can be prevented by the use of prophylactic penicillin to which the clostrida are uniformly sensitive (9). Bacteroides infection, after hysterectomy or lower intestinal operations, can be prevented by e.g. systemic metronidazole. In the absence of any such specific situation the antibiotic of choice must be one, or a combination, with as wide a spectrum of activity as possible. The relation between hospital use of antibiotics and the development of strains of micro-organisms resistant to them is such as to make it most desirable that the prophylactic use of antibiotics is guided by the microbiologist and directed in the way likely to give the best overall advantage.

PREVENTION

Some aspects of the prevention of sepsis have already been described ; sterilisation of materials, exclusion of dangerous carriers, disinfection of the hands, to which may be added the patients skin around the operation site and for operations on the gut, attempts to reduce the density of the intestinal flora.

Other considerations are : restriction of entry into the operating suite and room, in order to reduce the risk of a dangerous carrier being present ; exclusion of contaminated ward materials when the patient is brought in.

On the other hand there is a little indication and bacteriological evidence to discount, the suggestion that organisms from the floor play any part in the genesis of surgical sepsis. The value of masks is dabutable. The mouth flora are rarely implicated in infection and Staphylococcus aureus is dispersed from the skin of carriers, not from the upper respiratory tract. In addition friction at the mask edges may lead to increased dispersal of squames from the facial skin.

Used material is not usually heavily contaminated and presents less risk of carrying infection than do the staff. Where used material is contaminated with infected secretion then it may be easily and safely transported in sealed impermeable bags.

THE AIR OF OPERATING ROOMS

As a controversial issue this demands more detailed consideration. No convincing conclusions can be reached apart from a direct controlled clinical trial. The obstacles to this are considerable but a fully randomised prospective investigation of sepsis following total hip and knee joint replacement has recently been concluded (12).

Before discussing the results of this it may be useful to consider the methods and the extent, by which the air-contamination levels in the operating room can be reduced. First comes the number and activity of the persons in the room. Quite substantial differences can be made by limiting the staff to the minimum required and avoiding unnecessary activity. Secondly contaminated air from outside can be excluded by pressurised ventilation. When all this is done, however, the numbers of bacteria in the air are still considerable, an average value of some 150 bacteria-carrying particles/m^3 (aerobic cultivation) is usual.

It has been known for many years that the commonly worn cotton gown offers little or no barrier to the dispersal of micro-organisms from the body whether dry and into the air or wet by direct contact. As table 4 shows it is possible to obtain substantial reductions in dispersal by using different materials and designs.

Table 4.
OPERATING ROOM CLOTHING AND DISPERSAL OF SKIN BACTERIA[∅]

	Basic dress (loose weave)	Operating room clothing		Body-exhaust
		Cotton (loose weave)	Non-woven[⁑]	
Chamber tests	(100)			
Fabric alone	(100)	41	12	-
Simulated turbulent ventilation				
Gowns	(100)	67	40	7
Trouser suit		(100)[∇]	22(17)[§]	-
Simulated unidirectional ventilation				
Gowns	(100)	35	9	0.4
		(100)	26	1.1
Operating room : unidirectional ventilation[¶]				
Gowns		(100)	34	9
Trouser suit gown and hood		(100)	12	-

∅ Presented as relative values ;
⁑ Non-woven : felt of polyester and cellulosic fibres ;
∇ Actual values not significantly different from gowns ;
§ With elastic ankle closure ;
¶ Other sources in room, e.g. patient, contribute.

Compiled from Whyte et al (16) and unpublished, Lidwell et al (17).

The better performances of all the gowns in unidirectional flow ventilation is an obvious consequence of the large escape of dispersed organisms from the open bottom. The non-woven fabric is a fibrous mat which is strongly water repellent but has a good feel and is comfortable to wear, in contrast to the tightly woven fabrics of the "Ventile" type. When worn as a suit, with trousers fully snug around the ankle, dispersion is reduced between 5 and 10 fold compared with the convential cotton gown. This is almost as good as the results obtained with the ventilated whole-body-exhaust suit designed by Sir John Charnley.

Conventional ventilation systems produce a turbulent atmosphere in which the dispersed organisms are uniformly distributed over the whole room and removed gradually in a logarithmic fashion. In contrast unidirectional air flow systems remove them along the flow lines with a much increased efficiency. Such systems circulate a great deal more air and therefore, demand increased engineering investment. Several systems are illustrated in figure 1 and the resulting levels of airborne contamination shown in figure 2, wearing conventional cotton gowns or body-exhaust suit. It is clear that very large reductions in air-contamination levels can be attained.

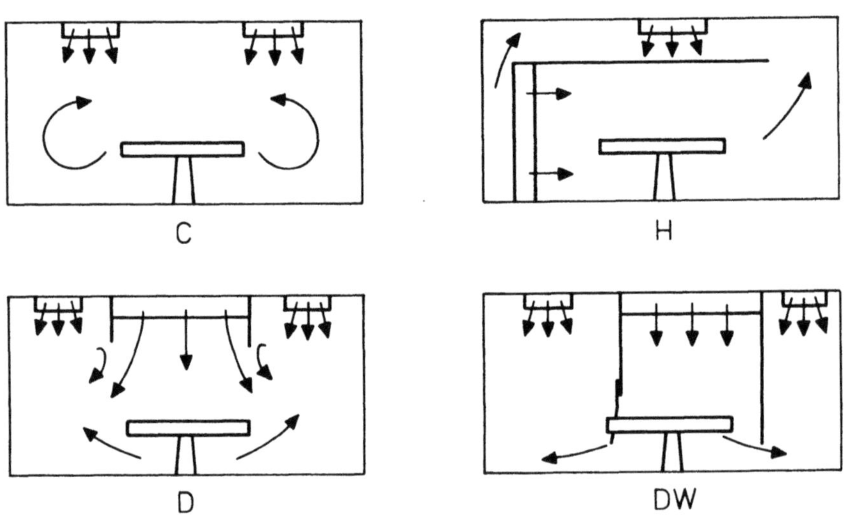

Figure 1. Types of ventilation.
C. Positive pressure turbulent supply.
H. Unidirectional horizontal flow.
D. Unidirectional downward air-flow, without walls below about 2 m. above the floor.
DW. Unidirectional downward air-flow, with walls to within about 15 cm. of the floor.

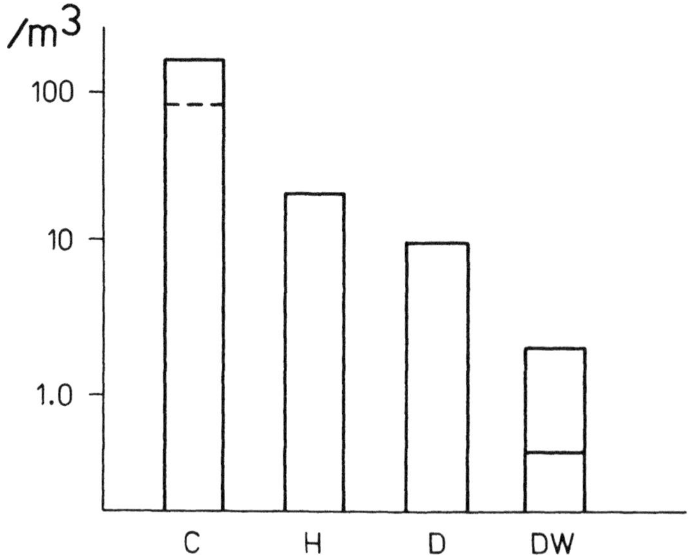

Figure 2. Average air-contamination levels obtained during surgical operations with different ventilation systems. Horizontal bars show the effect of wearing body-exhaust suits.
C. Turbulent supply.
H. Unidirectional horizontal air-flow.
D. Unidirectional downward air-flow, without walls below about 2 m. above the floor.
DW. Unidirectional downward air-flow, with walls to within about 15 cm. of the floor.

Does this have any effect on the incidence of sepsis. The British/Swedish study (12) involved over 8000 operation for hip of knee-joint replacement performed over a period of 3 years in 19 hospitals with each surgeon operating equally, without alteration in any other procedures, in a conventionally ventilated and in an ultraclean air environment. The average follow up time was between 2 and 2½ years. The results in relation to deep sepsis in the joint, severe enough to lead to reoperation, are summarised in table 5. There seems to be no doubt that there was less sepsis among the operations done in cleaner air.

Antibiotics were given prophylactically to about 2/3rds of the patients, but equally in conventional and ultraclean air conditions. Since antibiotic usage was closely related to hospital and surgeon the study does not provide a fully

Table 5.

EFFECT OF VENTILATION ON SEPSIS AFTER TOTAL JOINT-REPLACEMENT

	Percentage septic within 2 - 2½ years						
	Control series			Ultraclean air series			
Number of hospitals	Air contamination/m^3 ⁑	Clothing	Sepsis	Air Contamination/m^3 ⁑	Clothing	Sepsis	Sepsis ratio
10	158	Conventional	(36/1798) 2.0	7	Conventional	(16/1604) 1.0	2.0
10	133	Conventional	(27/2084) 1.3	0.5	Body exhaust ▽	(6/2133) 0.3	4.5

In brackets, number septic patients / number of operations
Data from multi-hospital investigation (12)
⁑ The air contamination levels are geometric mean values
▽ Includes also operations done in a plastic isolator

controlled examination of the influence of antibiotics. However, the apparent effect is very large and seems to operate independently of the effect of cleaner air. The combined effects of the two is shown in table 6 where the difference between conventional ventilation without antibiotics and the cleanest air situation combined with prophylactic antibiotics is dramatic.

Table 6.

COMBINED EFFECTS OF VENTILATION AND PROPHYLACTIC ANTIBIOTICS ON SEPSIS AFTER TOTAL JOINT-REPLACEMENT

	Percentage septic within 2-2½ years	
Ventilation	Without antibiotics	Prophylactic antibiotics
Control (turbulent)	(39/1161) 3.4	(24/2968) 0.8
Ultraclean		
Conventional clothing	(8/ 516) 1.6	(9/1279) 0.7
Body-exhaust suits ⁎	(5/ 544) 0.9	(1/1584) 0.06

Data from multi-hospital investigation (12).
In brackets, number septic patients / number of operations.
⁎ Includes operations done in a plastic isolator.

The conviction carried by these results is enhanced by the way they confirm other extensive but less well controlled studies. In addition a fully controlled doubleblind French study of antibiotics used in hip-joint replacement shows an almost identical benefit from antibiotic use (13).

QUANTITATIVE ASPECTS OF WOUND CONTAMINATION

Any environmental change in the operating room which influences the incidence of sepsis must do so by affecting the micro-organisms entering the wound during the operations and remaining there. Deposition from the air is illustrated in figure 3.

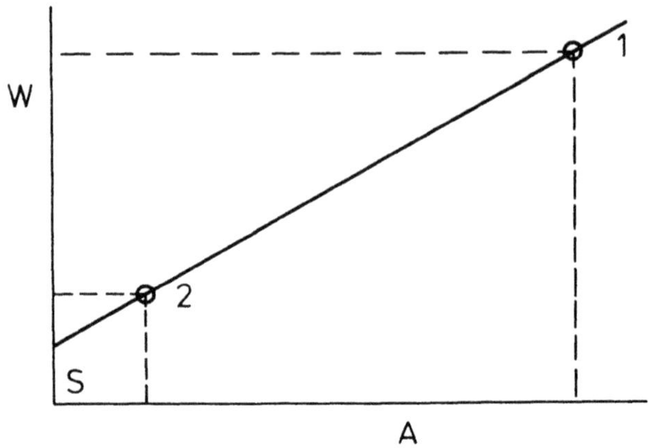

Figure 3. Sources of wound contamination.
Horizontal scale : A = air-contamination level.
Vertical scale : W = numbers of bacteria recovered by a wound wash-out.
S = contribution from non-airborne sources.

Sampling of the wound e.g. by washing out with fluid and culturing this, will then give relative values for the numbers under normal and ultraclean air conditions. From any two estimates, at different levels of air-contamination, it is possible to deduce the magnitude of the non-airborne contribution to the contamination of the wound (14). The results of such calculations suggest that, for the joint-replacement operations, this was about the same as that derived from air-contamination at a level of between 5 and $10/m^3$. This is close to the level of air-contamination reached by an ultraclean air system when conventional cotton gowns are worn. With body-exhaust suits, giving air-contamination levels around $1/m^3$, 90 % of the organisms reaching the wound will then come from non-airborne sources and the maximum attainable effect due to cleaner air would appear to have been reached. This study also suggests that the numbers of micro-organisms which fell directly into the wound were too few to account for t observed numbers recovered from it and that a large proportion of those found in the wound reached it indirectly ; e.g. from instruments etc., contaminated by exposure to the room air.

If the technical aspects of wound sampling can be improved this method of assessing the effect of changes in operating room practice on the risks of wound sepsis would seem to be a promising one. Evaluation in this way might approach the ultimate, clinical, evaluation.

The above results apply to deep sepsis in the joint, often manifesting itself months or even years after the operation for the implantation of the prosthesis. These operations are likely to be among the most susceptible to air-borne infection since they are carried out on a site free from risk of endogenous infection, are of relatively long duration and expose a large area. The extent to which the results may be applied in other fields of surgery remains to be determined.

In addition to deep sepsis in the joint the wounds were at risk to relatively superficial infection, such as is common to all types of surgery. When the records of the 8000 patients who received a joint implant are examined for superficial sepsis during the period of in patient stay a very different result appears, table 7.

Table 7.
WOUND SEPSIS (IN PATIENT), SURGEONS' ASSESSMENT **

	Ratio of incidence				
Degree of sepsis	C/UC	C/UC+	C/A11UC	NAB/AB	Rate in %
No evidence	0.98	1.23	0.99	0.98	91.6
Some evidence	1.08	1.20	1.08	0.86	3.3
Sepsis probable	1.13	1.25	1.14	1.42	4.1
Major sepsis	1.59	3.66	1.85	2.90	1.0
Number operated	3586	4164	8052 *	8052 *	

C = control, turbulent ventilation with conventional pattern clothing.
UC = ultraclean-air systems using convenional pattern clothing.
UC+ = body-exhaust suits in ultraclean-air system or Trexler plastic isolator.
NAB = no antibiotics given.
AB = prophylactic antibiotics given.

* Includes some control operations excluded from the balanced C/UC and C/UC+ comparisons.

** Data from multihospital investigation (12).

There is no evidence of any significant reduction in the incidence of this form of wound sepsis except in the relatively small number of cases of "major sepsis". These appear to be influenced by the conditions in the operating room and by the use of prophylactic antibiotics in a similar way to delayed sepsis deep in the joint and indeed they do, by definition, usually involve the deeper tissues. The value of cleaner air and antibiotics seems, therefore, to be restricted to a small minority, 10-15 % of cases of immediate post-operative wound sepsis. However, these are the most serious infections.

CONCLUSION

On the evidence so far available the maxim "don't touch the blade", with all it implies, seems to be one which covers most types of surgery. The evil in the air is, however, always present and makes itself apparent in at least one form of surgery, the total joint implant.

As a consequence of what has been said with regard to hand washing for the surgeon, the ease with which used materials can be safely removed at the end of the operation and the insignificance of floors as a route for microbial spread a rather simple plan for the operating suite would seem to combine efficiency, convenience and reasonable economy, figure 4.

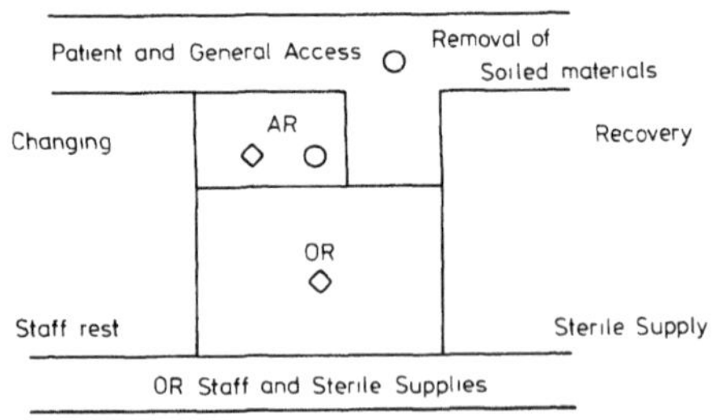

Figure 4. Schematic lay-out of operation suite.
OR = operating room.
AR = anaesthetic room.
◇ = air supply, filtered.
O = air extract.

The segregation of clean staff and sterile supplies from the, often busy, traffic of patient access and material disposal would seem to be rational although no investigation is likely to demonstrate any advantage with respect to surgical sepsis.

REFERENCES

1. Falkberget, J. 1940. Nattens Brød Vol. I, ch. 29 Aschehoug Oslo. Freely translated and condensed.
2. Meers, P.D., Ayliffe, G.A.J., Emmerson, A.M., Leigh, D.A., Mayon-White, R.T., MacKintosh, C.A., Stronge, J.L. 1981. Report on the National Survey of Infection in Hospitals, 1980. J. Hosp. Infection 2 : Supplement, Preface VIII.
3. M'tero, S.S., Sayed, M., Tyrrell, D.A.J. 1981. Quantitative studies on preventing the spread of micro-organisms in a hospital isolation unit. J. Hosp. Infection 2 : 317.
4. Lister, J. 1867. On the antiseptic priciple in the practice of surgery. Br. Med. J. II : 246.
5. Lister, J. 1890. An address on the present position of antiseptic surgery. Br. Med. J. II : 377.
6. Lowbury, E.J.L., Lilly, H.A., Ayliffe, G.A.J. 1974. Preoperative disinfection of surgeons hands : Use of alcolholic solutions and effects of gloves on skin flora. Br. Med. J. II : 869.
7. Rotter, M., Koller, W., Wewalka, G. 1980. Povidone iodine and chlorhexidine-gluconate-containing detergents for disinfection of hands. J. Hosp. Infection 1 : 149.
8. Working party 1972. Report of a joint working party on ventilation in operating suites. Medical Research Council and Department of Health and Social Security.
9. Parker, M.T. 1969. Postoperative clostridial infection in Britain. Br. Med. J. 3 : 671.
10. Blowers, R. 1962. Operating room practice. In : Infection in Hospitals. Eds Williams R.E.O. and Shooter R.A. Blackwell Oxford. 199.
11. Charnley, Sir J. 1979. Low friction arthroplasty of the hip Springer Verlag, Berlin, Heidelberg, New York.
12. Lidwell, O.M., Lowbury, E.J.L., Whyte, W., Blowers, R., Stanley, S., Lowe, D. 1982. The effect of ultra-clean air in operating rooms on deep sepsis in the joint after total hip or knee replacement: A randomised study. Br. Med. J. II : 10.
13. Hill, C., Flamant, R., Mazas, F., Evvard, J. 1981. Prophylactic cefazolin versus placebo in total hip replacement. Lancet. i : 795.

14. Whyte, W. 1982. J. Hosp. Infection in press.
15. Bengtsson, S., Hambraeus, A., Laurell, G. 1979. Wound infection after surgery in a modern operating suite. J. Hyg. (camb) 83 : 41.
16. Whyte, W., Vesley, D., Hodgson, R. 1976. Bacterial dispersion in relation to operating room clothing. J. Hyg. (camb) 76 : 367.
17. Lidwell, O.M., Mackintosh, C.A., Towers, A.G. 1978. The evaluation of fabrics in relation to their use as protective garments in nursing and surgery II. J. Hyg. (camb) 81 : 453.

GENERAL REFERENCES

Lister J. Baron 1899. Collected papers, Oxford the Clarendon Press.

Report 1962. Design and ventilation of operating-room suites for control of infection and comfort. Lancet II 45.

Report 1968. Aseptic methods in the operating suite. Lancet I 705, 763 and 831.

Control of Hospital Infection 2nd edtn 1981 ed. Lowbury E.J.L., Ayliffe G.A.J., Geddes A.M. and Williams J.D. London Chapman and Hall.

Design and utilization of operating theatres 1982 ed. Johnson I London Arnold in press.

COMMENTS ON THE OCCURRENCE AND PROPHYLAXIS OF SURGICAL INFECTIONS

R. K. J. KOUMANS

All surgical wound infections arise from one or both of two sources: the exogenous and/or the endogenous pathway of contamination. Different measures would seem necessery to block these pathways, corresponding roughly to rules of asepsis and antisepsis, respectively. A sutured wound is sealed with fibrin within a few minutes and, if properly handled, this fibrin forms an effective barrier against bacteria. This situation has four implications.

Postulate I: Surgical-wound infection is initiated at the time of surgery. A possible exception to this rule is the haematogenous "back door" to the wound, used by bacteria carried by the bloodstream, as shown experimentally by Howe (1). In surgery of the colon, episodes of systemic bacteremia occur in every third to fourth patient preoperatively (2). For surgical wounds, over-all infection rates are reported to fluctuate between 4% and 14%. These figures illustrate the magnitude of the problem, but are not helpful in an epidemiological investigation, unless operations are classified according to the estimated degree of contamination. In more than 60,000 operations, Cruse and Foord (3) found an over-all infection rate of 4.7%. The incidence was 1.5% in clean wounds as against 40.0% in heavily contaminated operations. An infection rate of 1.5% for clean wounds seems quite acceptable in current surgical practice, according to other reports and our own experience. It is of interest to note that a similar infection rate was reported by Brewer as early as 1915 (4). Evidently, endogenous sources are responsible for the formidable increase in wound infections in the heavily contaminated situation as well as for the less spectacular rates of infection in slight or moderately contaminated categories. Thus, if we wish to investigate the influence of exogenous pathways of contamination, these categories are no avail. This leads to:

Postulate II: Studies on exogenous (e.g., airborne) infection, must be done in series of "clean" (category I) wounds. This approach encounters two main problems. First, in view of the low infection rate, large numbers of clean operations have to be studied prospectively to permit valid conclusions. Secondly, if a clean wound becomes infected it does not mean automatically that exogenous micro-organisms are involved. Although aerial contamination has been implicated ever since the time of Lister, we still have no precise data on the number of wound infections resulting from airborne transmission versus other (endogenous or exogenous) sources. In a modern operating room with an air-conditioning system providing adequate input of filtered air and stringent aseptic discipline, the rate of exogenous infections can be kept at an almost negligible level, while endogenous routes of contamination remain essentially unaffected. On the other hand, available -- albeit possibly controversial -- evidence (5,6) points to the following:

Postulate III: Three out of every four infections in clean surgical wounds are caused by endogenous micro-organisms. Thus, to reduce the infection rate in clean surgery further, sophisticated methods for the prevention of airborne contamination are of limited avail, and peroperative antibiotic prophylaxis is indicated. This certainly appears to hold for cases where wound infection spells disaster, as in implant surgery.

The impact of prophylactic antibiotics can be studied best in a situation where wound contamination is unavoidable, for instance is surgery of the large bowel. In this contex I would like to briefly summarize our ouwn experience in this field. These data have been collected from the work of my former resident, Chris Ulrich (7). Initially, in a prospective blind pilot study started in the second half of 1976, we tried to assess the value of per-operative antibiotics (clindamycin and kanamycin) versus placebo in elective colorectal surgery. It must be kept in mind here that at that time the issue of antibiotic prophylaxis in colon surgery was still a matter of debate. When the 50th patient had entered the study, the code was broken. Since the wound infection rate was 66.7% in the controls versus 8% in the treated group ($p < 0.0005$), further study along these lines was ethically unjustifiable.

We then started a second (again prospective, randomized, and blind) study to find out whether a single pre-operative dose of clindamycin and kanamycin was as effective as a double (16 hr) or triple (24 hr) dose regimen. This group comprised 110 patients. Although the patients on a triple dose had fewer infections (16.2%) than those on a double dose (22.9%) or single dose (26.3%), the difference was not statistically significant.

At the same time, we performed a study on the efficacy of 24-hr prophylaxis with kanamycin/clindamycin versus kanamycin/cephalothin in emergency large-bowel surgery. The patients receiving clindamycin, which is specifically effective against bacteroides contamination, seemed to fare better, but this group was too small (56 patients) to show statistical significance. However, analysis of a more uniform subgroup (35 patients) with perforated appendicitis, did show significance (11.8% versus 55.6% infection rate). The incidence of wound sepsis in this emergency situation still seemed unacceptably high, possibly due to the fact that antibiotic administration was started during the operation, at the time when soiling was encountered. Therefore, in our next study, patients scheduled for emergency bowel surgery received clindamycin and kanamycin as soon as laparotomy was decided on. During the operation, patients were assigned to one of three groups on the basis of: A) little or no contamination, B) localized peritonitis or soiling, and C) generalized peritonitis or massive contamination.

In group A antibiotics were discontinued; group B received triple-dose (24 hr) prophylaxis; and in group C antibiotics were continued therapeutically for 5 days. In groups A (20 patients) and B (17 patients) no wound infection occurred. In group C (21 patients) the infection rate was 28.6%. These results compare favourably with those of the preceding study as well as with data in the literature, and perhaps reflect adequate concentration of antibiotics at the tissue level at the time when contamination took place. A vast amount of evidence has been accumulated in favour of per-operative antibiotic prophylaxis when macroscopic wound contamination is apt to occur. Extrapolation of the results to "clean" surgery, where microscopic contamination is involved, appears permissible. In fact, this is now commonly considered de rigeur in cardiovascular and orthopedic surgery when foreign material is implanted. Ultimately, surgeons will have to accept the fact that the objective of sterile surgery is Utopian.

Postulate IV: Bugs will continue to outsmart men. While striving to keep bacterial densities in our surgical wounds as low as possible, we may have to boost host defenses with antibiotics briefly but at the right time. Especially in cases where septic complications will compromise the results of our operations, the well-being of our patients, and/or the economic resources of both the patients and the community. We will then have to balance these interests against the risks of wide-spread -- albeit short-term -- use of potent, broad-spectrum antibiotics.

REFERENCES

1. Howe, C.W. 1968. Experimental wound sepsis from transient bacteremia. Surg. Gynec. Obstet. 126: 1066.
2. Burton, R.C. 1972. Gram-negative bacteraemia colonic rectal surgery. Med. J. Aust. 59 I: 367.
3. Cruse, P.J., Foord, R. 1980. The epidemiology of wound infection. A 10-year prospective study of 62939 wounds. Surg. Clin. North. Am. 60: 27.
4. Brewer, C.E.J. 1915. Studies in aseptic technique; with a report of some recent observations at the Roosevelt Hospital. JAMA 44: 1369.
5. Walter, C.W. 1979. The surgeon and postopertive wound infection. Arch. Surg. 114: 769.
6. Moggio, M., Goldner, J.L., McCollum, D.E., Beissinger, S.F. 1979. Wound infections in patients undergoing total hip arthroplasty. Ultraviolet light for the control of airborne bacteria. Arch. Surg. 114: 815.
7. Ulrich, C. 1981. Short term systemic antibiotic prophylaxis in colorectal surgery. Thesis, University of Leiden, The Netherlands.

DISCUSSION EDITED BY R.K.J. KOUMANS

Brouwer: I have a question for Dr. Koumans: Which drugs do you recommend for prophylaxis in large-bowel surgery? A combination of an aminoglycoside and clindamycin or a cephalosporin and metronidazole? Why do you prefer one combination to the other?

Koumans: After these studies were concluded about two years ago, we participated in a multicentre study to compare an aminoglycoside and metronidazole versus aminoglycoside and clindamycin. Only patients undergoing emergency large-bowel operations, in whom Bacteroides fragilis was cultured after contamination of the peritoneal cavity had occurred, were admitted to the study. No significant differences were observed between the two groups. Clindamycin and metronidazole appeared equally effective in preventing anaerobic septic complications. Because of the side effects of clindamycin, we now use metronidazole against anaerobes. With respect to the aerobes we originally chose kanamycin, because there is incomplete cross-resistence between that drug and the other clinically more valuable aminoglycosides and we did not want to run the more or less theoretical risk of inducing gentamicin- or tobramycin-resitant strains. After completing these studies, however, we switched to gentamicin because of its lower toxicity. So our preferred prophylactic combination is now metronidazole and gentamicin. Recently, we started another study along the same lines, to compare this double drug regime with a single-drug moxalactam prophylaxis.

Brouwer: Do you change the antibiotics according to sensitivity tests after you receive the bacteriological reports?

Koumans: We do not. As a matter of fact, we use a 24-hour triple dose prophylaxis and the laboratory results only come in later. However, when we encounter severe contamination or extensive periotonitis at operation, we continue the same drugs for five days. I am not wholly convinced, from the point of view of antimicrobial policy, that this is wise. Theoretically, once you decide to switch from prophylaxis to treatment it is preferable to change your drug combination too. Perhaps someone in the audience would like to comment?

van Furth: I think that a change would indeed be wise.

van der Meer: I would like to ask Dr. Lidwell if he can give us some information on late infections in total hip arthroplasties under the various regimens. For instance, is there an effect of antibiotic prophylaxis on the rate of late infections?

Lidwell: My data concern delayed deep infections only. They were collected from the records of those patients who had to have a re-operation. There was no significant difference between the clean-air systems or antibiotics with respect to the time when infections became manifest. There is of course evidence that haematogenous infections do occasionally occur in these situations, but they usually present themselves late and run a protracted course. One reason why we limited our follow-up period was that we though we could better evaluate the effect of these systems by not continuing too long, when haematogenous infections might play a bigger part and confuse the picture.

Mouton: I would like to ask Dr. Lidwell if he has any experience with the wound wash-out technique in neurosurgery. In craniotomies, after thorough decontamination of the scalp, high numbers of propionic bacteria and Staphylococcus epidermidis can be cultured from the incision, even where cultures of material from the skin surface before incision were negative. We have tried all sorts of measures to eliminate this flora, but have not succeeded. On the other hand, we have been unable to establish any relationship between the results of wash-out cultures and the occurrence of infection.

Lidwell: The answer to your first question is simple: I have no experience with bacteriological sampling in neurosurgical operations at all. I am not quite clear about your second question, concerning the skin organisms.

Mouton: Washing-out of the incision usually yields a lot of micro-organisms, although before incision the skin is quite sterile. Apparently, the bacteria arise from deep-seated skin appendages which are not reached by the disinfectants, for instance iodine.

Lidwell: I do not think that you ever were able to sterilize anyone's skin.

Mouton: Not completely, I agree.

Lidwell: There always remain bacteria in the deeper layers of the skin. Bacteriological studies of surgeons' hands after scrubbing demonstrate clearly that initially counts are very low. But within say 10 or 20 minutes, counts rise again as the skin surface becomes re-colonized from deeper down.

Mouton: That is certainly true, but bacterial density by re-colonization is especially high in the scalp, probably much higher than any contamination by air.

Lidwell: This is probably so. Another thing is that since the skin flora is mostly anaerobic, you will even get much higher counts if you culture anaerobically as well. On the other hand, contrary to some people's ideas, anaerobic organisms are also present in the air; they are not killed by floating in an oxygen-containing atmosphere. If you sample appropiately you will find as many skin anaerobes in air as aerobes.

Rubin: I think we have had a very fascinating discussion on bacteriology and the role of antimicrobial agents. I would just like to point out that we must also take host factors into account. Particularly what the surgeon does to the host. It has been well demonstrated in a variety of studies that obesity, duration of surgery, but particularly haemorrhage in the wound, play a significant role, and this last factor I think may well lead to a different approach to the problem of wound infection. There is a fascinating recent report of experiments in a rodent model, where haptoglobin was introduced into wound haematoma, obviously to bind haemoglobin and thus affect its availability as growth factor for bacteria. Wound infection rates were markedly decreased. So possibly rethinking about host factors will lead to alternatives in terms of prevention of wound infection, haptoglobin being perhaps one factor to be considered.

Goldmann: For the last ten years the neurosurgeons have kept requesting our operating committee to authorize the installation of ultraviolet lights to reduce the sepsis rate in neurosurgery. The cooperative study on this subject, though flawed, did show an effect of ultraviolet light in reducing neurosurgical infections. One of the interesting things in that study was the difference between organisms isolated from the air and those recovered from the wounds. I just wondered, Dr. Lidwell, if in your study the organisms isolated from the air bore any relationship to those recovered from the wound at the close of surgery or from infections later on?

Lidwell: That is not an easy question to answer. Generally speaking, the organims recoverd from the air, from the wounds, and from infections, are skin commensals of one sort or another. Groups in Glasgow and from Colindale Laboratories are attempting to do full indentification of strains from the different sources. So far, they have not fully reported. What I heard last from the Colindale people was that the strains recovered from the wash-out bore no clear relation to the strains from the patient's skin. The Glasgow people made a rather similar comment.

Goldmann: To put you in my place just for one second: six months from now those same neurosurgeons or the orthopaedic surgeons will come back to me and say: "Ha, ha, we don't want ultraviolet lights any more, we want this isolator system". What would you be prepared to say?

Lidwell: In hip-surgery my results appear to demonstrate that in the great majority of the cases bacterial contamination of the wound at the end of operation has arrived there via the air. Now, these wounds are very large, and are exposed for a very long time. I don't know neurosurgical operations would compare on a sort of area-time scale.

Goldmann: The wounds are much smaller and surgery takes about the same length of time.

Lidwell: Well, that would to some extent lower the contribution of airborne contamination in your system. But I think you also have to relate the answer to this question to what your infection problem is. If you are getting almost no infections, you will not have the same incentive as you would in dealing with the kind of situation in which we were when these studies were started, with infection rates round 10%. With reference to ultraviolet light, this has been perennial controversy. As you undoubtedly are well aware, as perennial as your question.

NOSOCOMIAL INFECTIONS IN COMPROMISED HOSTS

L. S. YOUNG

INTRODUCTION

Patients with impaired host defenses are clearly the most vulnerable for developing nosocomial infections. In spite of this generally acknowledged fact there has been a paucity of focused prospective epidemiologic studies of infections disease epidemiology in immunocompromised subjects. Most clinical studies emanate from large hospital centers that summarize the experience with a series of infections, e.g. Pseudomonas bacteremia, Aspergillus pneumonia etc. with limited insight into the factors which have concerned epidemiologists for much of the last two decades. Large nationwide nosocomial surveillance programs have not focused on immunosuppressed patients and failed to provide us with disease specific attack rates despite the fact that such patients are at increased risk (1). At the introduction of a recent international symposium on nosocomial infection Brachman of the U.S. Center for Disease Control states : "host factors such as the advanced age of patients in the presence of chronic diseases reduce resistance to infection" (2). No mention is made, however, of the problems of infection in recipients of organ transplants, individuals receiving chronic immunosuppressive or acute cytotoxic therapy and the very considerable problem of infection in patients with neoplastic diseases.

Studies of nosocomial infections, particularly those emphasizing multi-hospital surveillance tend to arrive at large over-all figures for infection incidence by service and by site/pathogen relationships, but few of these analyses have assessed the most critical variables in determining susceptibility to infection such as underlying disease and therapeutic intervention which impairs host resistance to infection. This commentary on nosocomial infections in compromised hosts might be expanded into a comprehensive treatise on the major types of infections that are likely to be encountered in the hospital setting. This is clearly beyond my scope and the reader is referred to comprehensive texts that have addressed themselves to this subject (3, 4), two recently published international symposia (5, 6), and a recent review (7). What I propose to highlight in these remarks is the nature of certain problems that one faces when one works in this field and some of the central issues that have been raised in the management of nosocomial infections in impaired hosts, particularly those of prevention and the cost-effectiveness of preventive measures.

METHODOLOGIC PROBLEMS

The basis of epidemiology is to establish a framework for analysis of certain observations. Very often this involves statistical comparisons. As has been pointed out by Freeman and McGowan, time is the important variable in any of these epidemiologic analyses (8), yet it must be remembered that with nosocomial infections that involve immunosuppressed patients, many patients develop repeated episodes of infections. The chronicity of predisposing host factors creates a situation where the same patients reappear over and over again with old or new infections. This creates problems in the interpretation of rates, and calls for the evolution of new analytical techniques. Thus, cohort studies which select groups of similar patients subjected to different variables are virtually impossible to carry out in compromised hosts. If one looks at leukemia treatment services for instance, the chemotherapeutic protocols that are used usually ensure equivalent exposure to certain risk factors. No clinical cancer chemotherapy unit would choose "to dilute" its patient population by using two or more protocols for treating the same underlying disease. The use of the case/control technique has become quite popular in studying outbreaks of disease and has led to crucial epidemiologic associations when field epidemiologists have faced challenging new problems, e.g. the initial studies of the toxic shock syndrome. Some case/control studies are possible such as selecting or comparing a renal transplant patient to an individual with renal failure who is not transplanted, but this type of analysis may exaggerate the differences between the study population and the controls. Furthermore, suitable controls, even if they have underlying diseases of a similar nature, may be treated by different methods which have their own risk of infection (e.g. renal dialysis instead of transplantation). Prevalence studies have been criticized in the chronic disease areas for the reason that the same patients may develop a multitude of problems in due time. It is commonly observed, for instance, that a patient with hematologic malignancy will first experience pneumococcal or staphylococcal infection, which is then followed by gram-negative infection, which in turn is supplanted by an opportunistic fungal process. At any one time in the clinical course a prevalence figure may be derived for that particular disease, but it may be better to follow the sequential events with time. As has been pointed out, perhaps one of the most valuable approaches to assessing nosocomial infections and any effect of intervention or attempted control measures is examination of survivorship as determined by life table analysis. Using this statistical method however, it may be possible to miss subtle associations since survival alone may not reflect episodes of major severe infections.

To compound our problems with the technical approaches to analysis of infection in the compromised host is the issue of diagnosis. Although everyone would accept the premise that infections are very common in individuals who are pancytopenic, hypogammaglobulinemic and subjected to immunosuppressive therapy, what one often sees in reviews of infections occurring in the compromised host is the assumption that fever is synonymous with infection. Do febrile patients really have an infectious process that is hospital acquired and is the cause of this febrile symptomatology ? Often it is recognized that febrile patients have negative cultures, but respond to empiric antimicrobial therapy. How to evaluate such episodes poses a real challenge. Even more frustrating are those patients who have fever with "definite" signs of infection, e.g. lung consolidation, but from whom no causative pathogen is isolated. As is often the case, individuals may have lung infiltrates but less than agressive measures are used to diagnose their etiology. Clearly, the true incidence of some infections may be underestimated and it will be equally difficult to say that some preventative or control measures are really efficacious given this setting.

In most reviews of nosocomial infections, a figure of 5 % overall incidence has been quoted (6). This figure must be greater for patients with altered immunity but is likely to vary greatly depending on specific disease. Few patients proceed through a course of chemotherapy for acute leukemia without developing fever and some signs of infection but leukemics seem at greater risk than patients being treated for solid tumors.

One of the few studies showing differential risk of a specific infectious complication focused on a recent epidemic of nosocomial Legionnaire's disease, where it was shown that renal transplant recipients had approximately 11 times greater risk than other individuals in the hospital for developing Legionnaire's disease (9). We are in sore need of similar types of data where different populations with similar types of exposure have been compared for the risk of developing a specific infectious complication. As has been pointed out "denominator data" for analyzing infectious complications by underlying disease is missing in many reviews (7).

NOSOCOMIAL PATHOGENS AND EPIDEMIOLOGIC CONSIDERATIONS

Table 1 that accompanies this section is an attempt to summarize the important nosocomial pathogens in immunosuppressed hosts and relevent epidemiologic considerations. Aerobic bacteria still account for the great majority and gram-negative bacilli have been quoted as responsible for more than half and possibly three quarters of all nosocomial infections (10).

Table 1.
NOSOCOMIAL PATHOGENS AND EPIDEMIOLOGIC CONSIDERATIONS

Bacteria	Host resistance	Pathogen virulence	Environmental factors	Other factors
Staphylococcus aureus	++	+++	+	Foreign body
Staphylococcus epidermidis	-	-	-	Foreign body
Staphylococcus pneumoniae	++	+++	-	
Corynebacteria	-	-	-	Foreign body
Gram-negative rods	++	+	+	Foreign body
Legionella pneumophilia	++	+++	+++	
Fungi				
Candida sp.	++	+	-	Foreign body
Aspergillus sp.	+++	+	+++	
Zygomycetes	+++	+	+++	
Cryptococci	+++	+	+	
"Epidemic" mycoses	+++	+	+	
Viruses				
Hepatitis	++	+++	-	Transfusions
CMV	+++	++	-	Transfusions
Varicella zoster	+++	+	-	
Herpes simplex	++	+	-	
Parasites				
Pneumocystis	+++		-	
Toxoplasma gondii	+++	+	-	
Strongyloides stercoralis	++	+	-	

This is probably true for the immunosuppressed host with possibly one exception : the apparent increase in Staphylococcus epidermidis and corynebacterial infections in the last few years that have been mainly associated with the use of indwelling intravascular catheters. Staphylococcus aureus is still a problem on surgical services but as an overall cause of bacteremia is less common than gram-negative bacilli. S. epidermidis and corynebacterium have little intrinsic virulence and compromised host resistance does not appear to be a major predisposing factor. These organisms are rarely significant pathogens unless there is a foreign body such as a vascular catheter in place. With Legionella pneumophilia host resistance is an important variable relating to disease incidence, the pathogen appears to be more virulent than ordinary gram-negative bacilli and environmental factors are extremely important in transmission. In contrast, Streptococcus pneumoniae which can be the cause of fulminant septicemia in the compromised host, may also appear as a life threatening pathogen in patients outside of the hospital whose underlying disease (such as Hodgkin's disease) has remitted.

Following the bacteria, perhaps the second major group of important pathogens are those organisms designated as opportunistic fungi. Nonetheless, in certain parts of the United States where natural environmental exposure to epidemic mycotic infections such as histoplasmosis, blastomycosis and coccidioidomycosis occurs, the immunosuppressed host may develop reactivation of an infection which had been previously contained while the host was healthy. Candida species leads the list of opportunistic fungal pathogens, particularly when abetted by a foreign body such as an indwelling venous or bladder catheter. Aspergillus species as well as the zygomycetes are commonly found in the environment and environmental factors probably play an important role in transmission. The role of the host is paramount in susceptibility to fungal infection and although each of the fungal pathogens listed has some virulence, it would be rare to see these clinical infections unless host defenses were compromised in some manner.

It has been estimated that viral infections probably account for less than 5 % of the nosocomial infections that occur in the United States (11). In the past hepatitis has received the most attention, particularly the infections that are transmitted via transfusions. That risk may be diminishing but a viral pathogen of considerably greater significance in some immunosuppressed patients is the cytomegalovirus. This virus has been recognized as not only the cause of severe pyrexia but of an often fatal opportunistic pneumonia. The risk of varicella-zoster or herpes simplex infections has varied considerably from institution to institution. Generally, the mortality from these rather common viral nosocomial infections has been relatively low.

Among the parasites, the one pathogen that has attracted much attention in recent years has been Pneumocystis carinii. Few normal subjects seem to develop pneumocystosis unless they have received immunosuppressive therapy. Environmental factors appear to be of little importance in the parasitic infections and most if not all of these processes represent recrudescent infection.

SITE OF NOSOCOMIAL INFECTION

Table 2 is an attempt to assess the relative role of infections at specific sites as expressed in general reviews of nosocomial infection contrasted to that encountered in compromised hosts. Perhaps the most striking difference is with urinary tract infections. Many general reviews have concluded that the urinary tract accounts for as many as 40 % of nosocomial infections. With the exception of the renal transplant population and catheterized subjects the urinary tract probably accounts for no more than 5 % of serious nosocomial infections in neutropenic subjects. In a prospective study of gram-negative bacteremia in neutropenic subjects at UCLA, only 1 of 34 episodes could be associated with an urinary tract source (12).

Table 2.
SITE OF NOSOCOMIAL INFECTION

	General reviews	Compromised hosts
Urinary tract	40 %	5 %
Respiratory tract	20 %	30 %
Wounds	20 %	5 %
Skin, soft tissue, bones	10 %	30 %
Gastrointestinal "primary bacteremia"	> 10 %	< 30 %

Respiratory tract infections are an important component of nosocomial infections in both the general hospital population and in compromised hosts. Proportionally they may be slightly greater in compromised host, but unfortunately there are many problems in identifying the nature of such respiratory tract infections. By definition wound infections represent complications developing in a wound secondary to surgery. Recent surgery is common in general hospital populations, but relatively uncommon in compromised hosts. The figure of 30 % or almost one third for skin and soft tissue infections relates to the high incidence of catheter associated infections in compromised hosts. That figure appears high, but represents one of the major trends in recent years. In most studies of nosocomial infections the grastrointestinal tract as a source has been hard to evaluate. The etiologic category of "primary bacteremia" has been used by the Center for Disease Control in the United States to apply to bloodstream infections where no apparent source can be identified (1). However, in prospective studies that we and others have carried out, a correlation between gastrointestinal colonization and the type of organism that is isolated from bloodstream of neutropenic patients developing Klebsiella and Pseudomonas bacteremia has been noted (12). It is our feeling that most of these bacteremias listed as "primary", if investigated adequately, represent a bloodstream seeding from a gastrointestinal focus.

With that framework in mind, the next table attempts to outline the opportunity for control of nosocomial infections and compromised host by site of involvement (Table 3).

Table 3.

THE OPPORTUNITY FOR CONTROL OF NOSOCOMIAL INFECTION IN COMPROMISED HOST

Urinary tract	Not a major problem
Respiratory tract	Limited prophylaxis vs. pneumocystis
Wounds	Not a major problem
Skin	Major area for improvement
Gastrointestinal "primary bacteremia"	Major area for improvement

Evaluation of impact of control measures involves the issue of cost effectiveness.

Since urinary tract infections are not a major problem in compromised host, we would subscribe that no special effort is required here other than the careful urinary catheter management techniques that have been evolved and proposed by many workers. With regard to respiratory tract infection, a major problem exists in the areas of diagnosis, treatment and prevention. Some small progress has been made by the demonstration that effective prophylaxis against Pneumocystis carinii is possible with the routine use of trimethoprim/ sulfamethoxazole. Aside from this, anecdotal reports suggest the benefit of protected environments with laminar air flow for reducing respiratory fungal infections, but it is doubtful that these will reduce bacterial and viral respirating infection that result either from aspiration of upper airway contacts or reactivation of latent infection. Wound infections in immunosuppressed patients are not a major problem unless such patients have previously been to surgery and such subjects usually account for a small fraction of the inpatient population. The skin as a source of infection is, however, a major area for improvement. Better methods for minimizing catheter associated infections are still needed. Finally, the gastrointestinal tract as a source of primary bacteremia has been a source of many investigations. This potential source of infection may be controlled by suppressing the endogenous or exogenously colonizing gram-negative bacterial flora of the gastrointestinal tract (7).

CONTROVERSIAL ASPECTS OF NOSOCOMIAL INFECTION CONTROL

It is easy to recognize the problems, as summarized in the previous tables and to stipulate which areas are in need of improvement. It is clearly more difficult to evaluate control methods. Not only are better clinical studies needed but solid evidence must be presented of the cost/effectiveness of a specific form of intervention. I have listed in Table 4 the major areas controversy where studies have appeared to support or negate certain approaches.

Table 4.
CONTROVERSIAL ASPECTS OF NOSOCOMIAL INFECTION CONTROL

1. Control of antibiotics to reduce incidence of infection or limit emergence of resistance.
2. Augmentation of host resistance
   a. supplying exogenous granulocytes
   b. active immunization
   c. passive serotherapy.
3. Environmental control
   a. protective isolation
   b. protective environments.
4. Antimicrobial prophylaxis
   a. suppression of gastrointestinal flora
   b. antifungal agents (prophylaxis vs. therapy of difficult to diagnose invasive disease).

First, the value of control of antibiotics to reduce the incidence of infection or limit emergence of resistance has been assumed to be true by many workers. The problem of nosocomial infections has been easily blamed on indiscriminate use of antimicrobial agents. However, there is no evidence from any controlled, prospective study that I am aware of that the control of antibiotics in hospital settings actually reduces the incidence of infection or limits the emergence of resistance. In fact, the use of newer antibiotics to aggressively treat the first signs of infection in compromised hosts may well reduce emergence of resistance to older compounds as illustrated by the initial use of amikacin and its impact on gentamicin resistance in the hospital (14).

A far more appealing approach to nosocomial infection prevention in compromised hosts has been an attempt to correct the basic defect, namely to augment host-resistance. Unfortunately such approaches offer more promise than reality. Active immunization, as in the case of Pseudomonas immunization has been attempted by many workers and results are promising in certain areas such as thermal injury (15). On the other hand, active immunization of immunosuppressed patients is likely to have limited effects, as evidenced by the experience with pneumococcal immunization. Supplying exogenous granulocytes is intrensically appealing but the complications of such granulocyte transfusions has been sobering (16).

The twin subjects of environmental control and antimicrobial prophylaxis can be linked together. "Protective isolation" has not been shown to be superior to such measures as careful handwashing. The use of protected invironments incorporating laminar air flow appears to have reduced infection in several studies, yet alternative less costly methods could be equally effective (17). Antimicrobial suppression of the GI flora can reduce infection incidence but may lead to emergence of a more resistant bacterial flora (18).

CONCLUSIONS

There are no easy answers to the issues of nosocomial infection control in immunosuppressed patients. These individuals are at great risk and the accurate antemortem diagnosis of infection is often frustrating. Two areas can be identified as being amenable to greater efforts at nosocomial infection control : 1) infections of the skin and soft tissues, and 2) infections that may originate in and around the gastrointestinal tract. Respiratory infections remain one of the most difficult challenges that are faced in the management of the immunosuppressed patient. Many costly techniques, including granulocyte transfusions and laminar air flow units and some potentially dangerous techniques such as antimicrobial prophylaxis have been developed in an attempt to prevent disease. While there studies to support their efficacy, the issue of cost effectiveness has not been squarely faced. Additionally, the question of how much disease is actually preventable still needs to be tested in careful comparative prospective studies in high risk groups. It is doubtful, for instance whether the results obtained in prevention of infection in acute leukemia can be directly applied to other high risk groups such as those with burns or renal transplants. The challenge for those working in the area of nosocomial infections in the compromised host will be to use sound analytical epidemiologic tools and to demonstrate that some forms of active intervention not only are efficacious, but have an impact upon patient survival and are fully justifiable from the viewpoint of cost.

REFERENCES

1. Center for Disease Control. March 1981. National nosocomial infection study report, 1978. Center for Disease Control, Atlanta, Georgia.
2. Brachman, P.S. 1981. Nosocomial infection control : An overview. Rev. Inf. Dis. 3 : 640.
3. Rubin, R.H., Young, L.S. (eds). 1981. The Clinical Approach to Infection in the Compromised Host. New York. Plenum Publishing, 653.
4. Grieco, M.H. (ed). 1980. Infection in the Abnormal Host. New York : Yorke Medical Books, 1035.
5. Dixon, R.E. (ed). 1981. Symposium on Nosocomial Infections. Am. J. Med. 70 : 379-472, 631-744, 899.
6. Sacks, T., McGowan, J.E. Jr. (eds). 1981. International Symposium on Control of Nosocomial Infection. Rev. Inf. Dis. 3 : 635.
7. Young, L.S. 1981. Nosocomial infections in the immunocompromised adult. Am. J. Med. 70 : 398.
8. Freeman, J., McGowan, J.E. Jr. 1981. Methodologic Issues in Hospital Epidemiology II. Time and Accuracy in Estimation. Rev. Inf. Dis. 3 : 668.
9. Bock, B.V., Kirby, B.D., Edelstein, P.H., et al. 1978. Legionnaire's disease in renal transplant recipients. Lancet 1 : 410.

10. Egoz, N., Michaelli, D. 1981. A program for surveillance of hospital-acquired infections in a general hospital : A two year experience. Rev. Inf. Dis. 3 : 649.
11. Valenti, W.M., Menegus, M.E., Hall, C.B., Pincus, P.H., Douglas, R.G. Jr. 1980. Nosocomial viral infections I. Epidemiology and significance. Infection Control 1 : 33.
12. Young, L.S., Meyer, D.V., Winston, D.J., Feig, S.A., Gale, R.P. and UCLA Bone Marrow Transplant Group. 1979. Gram-negative rod bacteremia : epidemiologic aspects in markedly neutropenic subjects and approaches to immune prophylaxis. In Vanderwaaij D. and Verhoef J. (eds), New Criteria for Antimicrobial Therapy. Amsterdam, Excerpta Medica (no. 447), 30.
13. Hughes, W.T., Kuhn, S., Chaudhary, S., Feldman, S., Verzosa, M., Aur, R.J.A., Pratt, C., Eorge, E.L. 1977. Successful chemoprophylaxis of Pneumocystis carinii pneumonitis. N. Eng. J. Med. 297 : 1419.
14. Price, K.E., Kresel, P.A., Rarchione, L.A., Siskin, S.B., Karpow, S.A. 1981. Epidemiological studies of aminoglycoside resistance in the USA. J. Antimicrob. Chemother. 8 (Suppl. A) 89.
15. Young, L.S., Pollack, M. 1980. Immunologic approaches to the prophylaxis and treatment of Pseudomonas aeruginosa infection. In Sabath L. (ed) : Pseudomonas aeruginosa. Berne : Hans Huber, 119.
16. Young, L.S. 1982. Prophylactic granulocytes in the neutropenic host. Ann. Int. Med. 96 : 240.
17. Berdischewsky, M., Young, L.S. 1979. Infectious complication of neoplastic disorders and their management. In, Franklin E.C. (ed), Current Topics in Immunology, New York : Elsevier North Holland Press, 307.
18. Dekker, A.W., Rozenberg-Arska, M., Sixma, J.J., Verhoef, J. 1981. Prevention of infection by trimethoprim-sulfamethoxazole plus amphotericin B in patients with acute nonlymphocytic leukemia. Ann. Int. Med. 95 : 555.

ANTIBIOTIC STRATEGY IN MYELOCOMPROMISED PATIENTS

J.W.M. VAN DER MEER, W.E. FIBBE, and P.J. VAN DEN BROEK

Many studies have shown that neutropenic patients are prone to develop infections caused by nosocomial microflora resistant to many antimicrobial drugs. These micro-organisms have usually colonized the patient prior to the the onset of the infection (1,2). Previous broad-spectrum antimicrobial therapy is probably one of the main factors contributing to this colonization. Thus, in such patients each course of antimicrobial therapy creates potential problems. Unlike many physicians who start broad-spectrum antibiotic treatment at the first spike of fever in a neutropenic patient, we give preference to a more conservative approach (3-5). We do not believe that immediate antibiotic treatment is necessary in all febrile neutropenic patients. We try to judge on clinical grounds whether infection is likely or not, and whether antimicrobial therapy should be instituted immediately. If infection seems unlikely, we withold antibiotic treatment and keep a careful watch on the patient. The algorithm we use is represented in chapter 10.

If antimicrobial therapy is required, we do not give a standard regimen of antimicrobial drugs, but tailor the treatment according to the criteria given in Table I.

To our knowledge the results obtained with this approach have not been compared with those of the more agressive approach, i.e., broad spectrum "empiric" antimicrobial therapy. The reasons for choosing for the latter approach are mainly anecdotal.

Table I.

PARAMETERS FOR THE CHOICE OF ANTIBIOTICS IN MYELOCOMPROMISED PATIENTS WITH A PRESUMED INFECTION

1. Duration of hospital stay
2. Previous use of antibiotics
3. General condition
4. Stage of underlying disease
5. Results of surveillance cultures
6. Possible localization of infection
7. Results of microbiological investigations (Gram staining, cultures)
8. Prevalent microflora in the hospital

The advantages of the more conservative approach characterized by limitation of the use of antibiotics, are obvious:

1. There is less interference with diagnosic procedures.
2. There is, as already mentioned, less disturbance of the microflora of the patient and the environment, wich in turn reduces subsequent colonization with multiple-resistant bacteria and fungi.
3. Costs are lower.
4. Drug toxicity occurs less often.

The question is, of course, whether our approach leads to greater mortality. Although we have not performed a controlled trial, we have collected data prospectively in our hospital during 1981. The number of evaluated patients are given in the algorithm (Fig. 1).

It should be kept in mind that this analysis only concerned granulocytopenic episodes (< 500 granulocytes/mm^3) with fever higher than 39.5°C (measured in the axilla). Of the 46 granulocytopenic patients with fever, 29 were judged to have an infection and treated accordingly. In 18 of these patients a causative micro-organism was found, and in 11 patients the cause of the infection remained unknown. Of the 18 with an identified

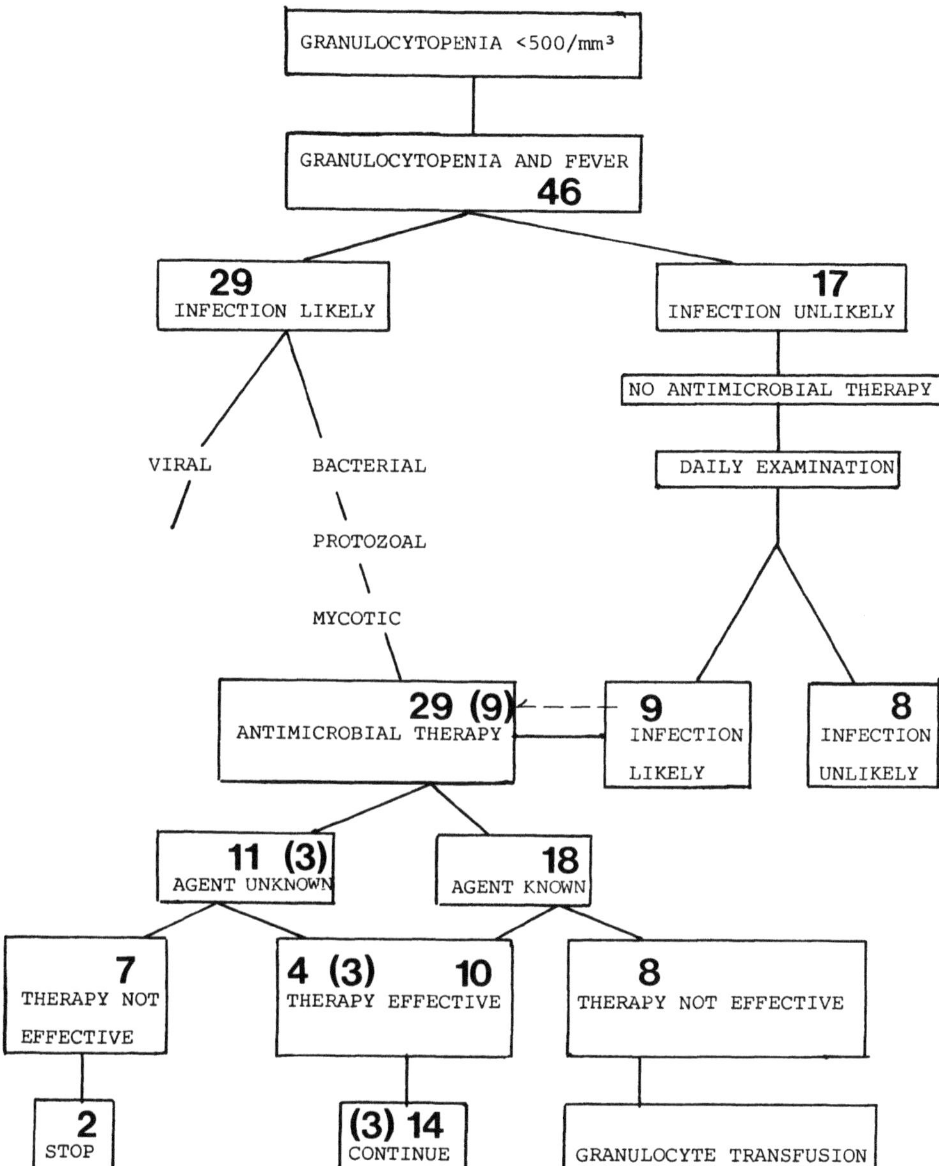

Fig. 1. Algorithm for management of granulocytopenic patients with fever; data of a prospective study are filled in. Between parentheses the numbers of patients in whom infection was initially thought to be unlikely are given.

micro-organism, therapy was effective in 10 and was not effective in 8. Of the 11 without a known micro-organism therapy was judged effective in 4, and ineffective in the remaining 7. Of the 17 patients judged as having not a serious infection, 9 were found in the follow up to have an infection, and in 6 of the latter patients a causative micro-organism was found. Of these 6 cases therapy failed in only one (because of weekend service there was a delay in the institution of appropriate antimicrobial therapy in this patient).

Of our 46 neutropenic, febrile patients, 14 died (30.4%). In considering such mortality figures, it is important to take the stage of the underlying disease into account. Of these 14 patients, no fewer than 9 were refractory to anti-leukemic treatment. Among the five non-refractory patients, one death (possibly preventable) has already been mentioned; another of this group was a 64-year-old woman who developed peritonitis (with sterile blood cultures) and one proved to have sufferd from legionellosis but had not responded to erythromycin therapy. One patient was admitted in septic shock (E. coli) and died. The fourth patient died, despite adequate antimicrobial therapy, of bacteremia originating from the gastro-intestinal tract.

From the present findings it may be concluded that it seems possible to use clinical grounds to select those patients who need immediate antibiotic therapy, and that a restricted patient-tailored use of antibiotics can be applied in myelocompromised patients. The outcome is almost entirely dependent on the stage of the underlying disease.

REFERENCES

1. Schimpff, S.C., Young, V.M., Creene, W.H., et al. 1972. Origin of infection in acute non-lymphocytic leukemia. Significance of hospital acquisition of potential pathogens. Ann. Int. Med. 77: 707.
2. Meyer, D.V., Winston, D., Young, L.S., et al. 1980. Surveillance cultures in immunosuppressed patients - What do they mean? In: Current chemotherapy and infections disease. Eds J.D. Nelson and C. Grassi. American Society for Microbiology. Washington. 1436.
3. Nauta, E.H., Furth van, R. 1975. Infection in immunodepressed patients. The approach to diagnosis and Treatment. Infection. 3: 202.

4. Meer van der, J.W.M., Alleman, M., Boekhout, M. 1979. Infectious episodes in severely granulocytopenic patients. Infection 7: 171.
5. Broek van der, P.J., Meer van der , J.W.M. 1979. Antimicrobial therapy in the myelo- and immunocompromised patient. Neth. J. Med. 22: 118.

DISCUSSION EDITED BY J. W. M. VAN DER MEER

Roord: Dr. van der Meer, were autopsies performed on the patients that died without a known infectious agent? If so, were there any signs of infection at autopsy?

van der Meer: Of these five cases, an autopsy was performed in one and the findings confirmed the clinically suspected diagnosis disseminated candidasis.

Roord: You had nine deaths in the group with a known agent. Did these patients receive granulocyte transfusions?

van der Meer: The indication we apply for granulocyte tranfusion is a persistent proven bacterial infection in patients with less than 100 granulocytes/mm^3. However, if a patient is considered haematologically refactory, we do not transfuse granulocytes. In the present series only one patient received granulocyte transfusions.

Young: The data from several American centres on patients refractory to all forms of treatment show that more than half of these patients have disseminated fungal disease. If such patients have been on empiric amphotericin B or one of the imidazoles, it may no longer be possible to document the original infection at autopsy. This again reflects the challenge involved in understanding the epidemiology of infection in these patients, and it is something we must recognize when we attempt to do epidemiologic analysis either retrospectively or prospectively.

van der Meer: I agree. Another point, as you have pointed out elsewhere (Am. J. Med. 7: 398), is that the number of autopsies performed influences the observed incidence of say fatal aspergillosis. Nevertheless, with a rather high proportion of autopsies done, and taking our material together, we have seen very few aspergillus infections in our leukemia patients. I think there are two major explanations for this. First of all, for some geographic reason, there are fewer fungi (especially Aspergillus species) present in The Netherlands. The second explanation is, I think, although we have no evidence to support it, the conservative antibiotic policy.

Rubin: I would like to make two points. The first is to remind the audience that one should not lump all compromised patients together. There is a big difference between dealing with bone marrow transplantation of leukemia patients, patients with Hodgkin's disease undergoing intensive chemotherapy, and renal transplant patients. Secondly, I would definitely agree with Dr. van der Meer, where he pointed out that the decisions about "whether or not antibiotics are started" and "which regimen we choose" are dependent on the stage of the underlying disease. I think it is terribly important to use a time-table of expected infection. I will discuss this time-table in greater detail for the renal transplant patient (see Chapter 18), but I would suggest here that there is an expected time-table for each of these immunocompromised patients. Such a time-table becomes very useful in two ways: it becomes a guide to the clinician in the management of the individual patient when decision-making is necessary, and secondly, when you see exceptions to the time-table, it means that something is wrong. In our experience, exceptions to these time-tables may indicate an excess nosocomial hazard that we were not aware of beforehand.

BACTERIAL INFECTION IN THE CRITICALLY-ILL NEONATE

D.A. GOLDMANN

In the past decade there has been a rapid proliferation of regional neonatal intensive care units (NICUs) in the United States. There can be no doubt that the advances in intensive care offered in such units have permitted the survival of critically ill, very low birth weight babies who surely would have perished just a few years ago. Unfortunately, the recovery of many babies has been jeopardized by nosocomial infections, which have become a significant hazard of neonatal intensive care. In recent years there have been numerous fulminant, difficult-to-control outbreaks of nosocomial infection, often associated with considerable morbidity and high mortality rates (1-9). Whereas Staphylococcus aureus was the major nursery pathogen during the 1950's and 1960's, today's epidemics are usually caused by gram-negative bacilli such as Klebsiella, Enterobacter and Pseudomonas.

Explosive epidemics such as these make for exciting reading, and it is perhaps for this reason that they have been amply documented in the pediatric literature. Much less attention has been devoted to the risk of nosocomial infection when there is no epidemic in the nursery, but it has become clear that this risk is substantial. For example, a review of the nosocomial infection experience in the University of Utah Medical Center NICU revealed that 15.3 % of babies remaining in the nursery for at least 48 hours - or 12.0 % of all babies admitted to the NICU - developed nosocomial infections (10). Some of the infections were quite minor and did not require systemic antibiotic therapy, but the majority of babies had serious infections, including pneumonia, bacteremia and meningitis. The risk of nosocomial infection was significantly higher for very low birth weight neonates. The authors of this study speculated that the rather high rate of infection in their NICU was also due to the many invasive diagnostic and therapeutic procedures to which the babies were subjected, and they noted that the crowded conditions which prevailed in the nursery may have contributed to the nosocomial infection problem. However, no data were provided to support these hyptheses.

At the Children's Hospital Medical Center in Boston, we have performed a study to more closely examine the impact of host, therapeutic and environmental factors on the risk of neonatal nosocomial infection (11). The Children's Hospital NICU is a referral center which receives seriously ill patients from the entire New England area. Patients requiring major surgery are not usually admitted to the NICU and are cared for elsewhere in the hospital. Nosocomial infections were prospectively monitored from 1974 through 1978 by a trained infection control practitioner using standard definitions from the Centers for Disease Control which were adapted to the neonatal care setting (12). In general, infections were considered nosocomial if they were first noted more than two days after admission, but cases had to be analysed individually since peri-natally acquired infections sometimes do not appear until a number of days after birth. Neonates were considered to have bacteremia if they had one positive percutaneously-obtained blood culture and a compatible clinical picture, provided that they received specific antibiotic therapy. Neonates from whom the same organism was recovered in two consecutive blood cultures were considered to have bacteremia regardless of clinical presentation or therapy. These rather arbitrary criteria were necessary because our physicians were usually unable or unwilling to obtain more than one blood culture from tiny, possibly septic babies before starting antibiotic therapy. Our definition of pneumonia also was less than ideal because of the difficulty in distinguishing radiologically between the infiltrates of pneumonia and the pulmonary changes of respiratory distress syndrome and other disorders of the neonatal lung. Moreover, it was difficult to obtain adequate sputum samples without endotracheal intubation or lung puncture. Most of the patients who were given the diagnosis of nosocomial pneumonia had positive cultures of sputum obtained from an endotracheal tube in combination with compatible chest roentgenograms and clinical presentations. A few patients were judged to have pneumonia in the absence of adequate cultures because they had clinical and radiographic findings that were most consistent with bacterial pneumonia and received an appropriate course of antibiotic therapy. Definitions for other types of nosocomial infection did not require substantial modification. Nosocomial infections caused by viruses were not routinely monitored during the study period and were thus not included in this investigation. Necrotizing enterocolitis was not included unless it resulted in bacteremia or other frank infection meeting the above criteria.

The microbiology of the major nosocomial infections encountered during the study period is summarized in Table 1.

Table 1.

ETIOLOGIES OF MAJOR NOSOCOMIAL INFECTIONS IN THE NICU OF CHILDREN'S HOSPITAL MEDICAL CENTER, 1974-1978

Type of infection, organism	Number of infections
Bacteremia	
Klebsiella pneumoniae	10
Staphylococcus epidermidis	8
Staphylococcus aureus	4
Enterococcus	2
Escherichia coli	2
Acinetobacter sp.	1
Pseudomonas aeruginosa	1
Viridans streptococci	1
Torulopsis glabrata	1
Candida albicans	1
Meningitis	
Klebsiella pneumoniae	4
Escherichia coli	1
Staphylococcus aureus	1
Staphylococcus epidermidis	1
Torulopsis glabrata	1
Candida albicans	1
Pneumonia	
Pseudomonas aeruginosa	8
Pseudomonas cepacia	6
Klebsiella pneumoniae	4
Escherichia coli	2
Enterobacter sp.	2
Staphylococcus aureus	2
Acinetobacter sp.	1
No diagnostic culture obtained	4
Wound	
Klebsiella pneumoniae	1
Peritonitis	
Pseudomonas cepacia	1
Klebsiella pneumoniae	1
Osteomyelitis	
No diagnostic culture obtained	1
Urinary tract infection	
Escherichia coli	1
Proteus mirabilis	1

Note. Total number of bacterial isolates is greater than the total number of infections because multiple pathogens were isolated from some infections.

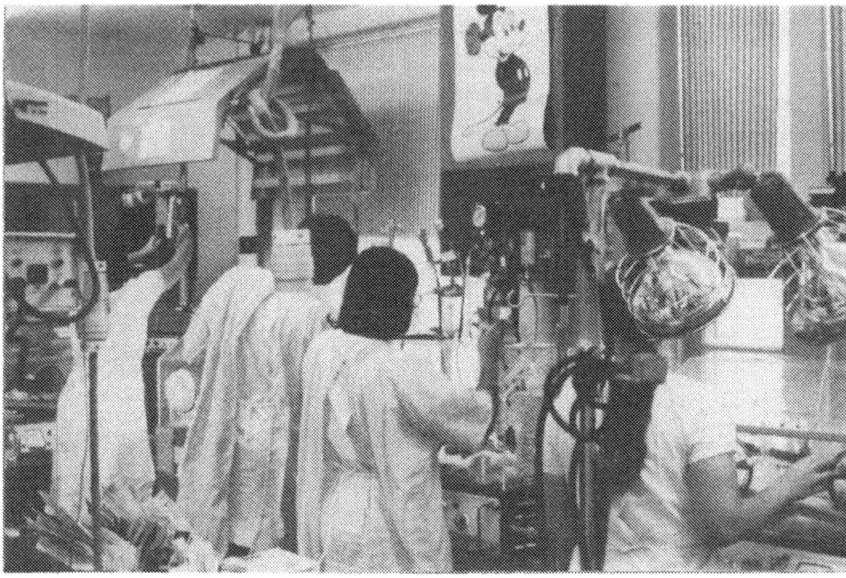

patients were unavailable) to 38 randomly chosen uninfected babies. All factors for which information was routinely recorded in the medical records were analyzed. For infected patients, consideration was limited to attributes and events that preceded the onset of nosocomial infection. To compare effects of variables with multiple levels of exposure (for example, duration of intravascular catheterization), each case was matched with a control patient whose duration of hospitalization was the same as the number of days the infected baby was hospitalized before infection was noted. This matching procedure was necessary because infected patients generally had considerably longer hospitalizations than the randomly chosen controls, so there was a greater opportunity for them to be exposed to potential risk factors.

The most glaring nosocomial infection risk factor was found to be low birth weight. The mean birth weight of infected babies was 1581 grams versus 2607 grams for comparison subjects. Linear trend analysis revealed a linear increase in the risk of major nosocomial infection with decreasing birth weight ($p < 10^{-8}$); the slope was 0.03 (95 % confidence interval, 0.02 - 0.04), which indicates that there was a 3 % increase in the risk of nosocomial infection for every 500 gram decrease in birth weight. Because of this striking effect of birth weight on infection risk, all subsequent comparisons were controlled for this variable by stratifying patients into very low, low and moderate birth weight groups. The additional risk factors which we were able to identify provided no surprises. They fell into four general categories : (1) diagnosis of patent ductus arteriosus and surgery (principally for ligation of patent ductus arteriosus) ; (2) measures required to maintain adequate oxygenation (endotracheal intubation and duration of intubation, high fractional concentration of inspired O_2, and high peak ventilatory pressure) ; (3) measures required to maintain intravascular volume and nutritional status (duration of umbilical artery catheterization, number of blood, plasma and albumin transfusions, and administration of hyperalimentation and lipid solutions ; and

(4) duration of antibiotic administration. Most of these risk factors tended to be found together in the sickest patients and were probably interrelated.

In February 1977 the NICU was relocated to a new facility with superior infection control design features (Figure 2).

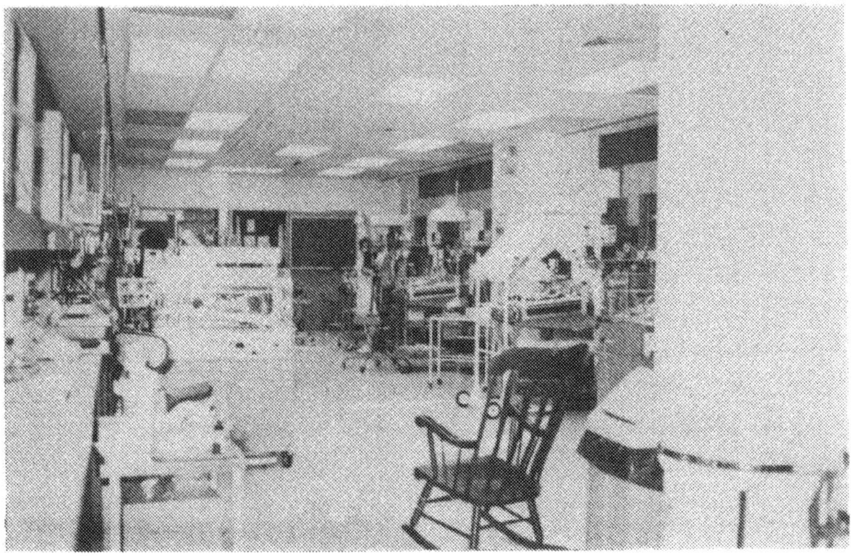

Figure 2. View of new nursery.

Although built to accommodate 16 neonates, only 12 babies were hospitalized in this "new nursery" during the study period. There was one large patient-care area which was divided by a chest-high partition that permitted cohorting of colonized or infected patients when necessary. A private room was available for patients who required respiratory precautions or complete isolation. Excluding this isolation room, the patient care area was 156 m^2, or 13.0 m^2 per neonate - a three-fold increase over the area of the old nursery. Ventilation was provided at 12 exchanges of air per hour through high-efficiency particulate air filters. Sinks were plentiful and conveniently located. Perhaps the most significant change was a 50 % increase in the nursing staff which permitted a natural cohorting system with one nurse caring for only two babies on most shifts.

Shortly after this move, there was a dramatic fall in the nosocomial infection rate. In the new nursery, only 0.9 % of the babies acquired a nosocomial infection. After stratifying patients in the old and new nurseries by birth weight, the decline in the infection rate was highly significant (Mantel-Haenszel relative risk, old nursery/new nursery 5.06, 95 % confidence interval 2.62 - 9.73). If only infants who remained in the NICU for more than 48 hours were included in the analysis, the fall was even more striking (relative risk, old nursery/new nursery 9.73, 95 % confidence interval 4.30 - 22.0).

Was the precipitous fall in the infection rate due to better staffing and an improved nursery environment, or were patients in the new nursery at less risk for nosocomial infection because they were not as ill as old nursery babies and required fewer invasive diagnostic or therapeutic procedures ? Could the decreased infection rate be attributed to changes in infection control procedures ? We concluded that what we have always taken for granted is, in fact, true - adequate staffing and environment can prevent nosocomial infection. We could identify no changes in infection control policy that coincided with relocation of the nursery, and the rate of infection in the rest of the hospital remained stable at 2.0 % for the entire study period. In addition, we performed a cohort study to determine whether new nursery patients had similar exposure to the risk factors for nosocomial infection which we had identified in the old nursery case-control study ; we discovered that new nursery babies tended to have a more intense exposure to these risk factors.

Almost everyone who had the opportunity to walk through our old nursery came away with the same explanation for the high rate of infection. Personnel simply did not have the time, facilities, or morale for practicing good infection control technique, particularly hand washing. Nursery staff repeatedly contaminated their hands with nosocomial pathogens while caring for colonized babies, forgot to stop at the sink and thus transmitted the pathogens to other critically ill, high risk patients.

In order to document neonatal acquisition of nosocomial pathogens in our old nursery, we obtained semiquantitative nose, throat, umbilicus and stool cultures from 63 babies every three days until discharge (14). To appreciate the abnormal colonization we observed in these NICU babies, it is helpful to review the evolution of bacterial flora in babies who do not require intensive care. Within the first few days of life, healthy, term babies develop a "normal" bacterial flora derived from contact with mother and the nursery environment. Alpha streptococci predominate in the throat and S. epidermidis in the nose and umbilicus. The stool flora of breast-fed babies includes large numbers (10^7 - 10^{10} cfu/gram) of Bifidobacteria (anaerobic lactobacilli) and smaller numbers of other anaerobes. Although E. coli is found in the stool of many newborns, it generally is overshadowed by the Bifidobacteria. Other gram-negative bacilli, such as Klebsiella and Pseudomonas are rarely cultured from the stool of breast-fed babies. The stool flora of formula-fed babies more closely resembles that of adults, although it is less varied. E. coli may outnumber the Bifidobacteria and Bacteroides, and other anaerobic bacteria are more prominent. Klebsiella, Pseudomonas and other aerobic gram-negative bacilli may be recovered from stool cultures, but they virtually never displace the E. coli.

The stool flora of babies hospitalized in our NICU developed in an entirely different fashion, perhaps in part as a result of the barrage of antibiotics most patients received, as well as the separation of neonates from their mothers. In our study, bacterial colonization was delayed at all sites cultured. After three days of hospitalization, almost one-third of the study patients had no growth from most cultures, and even stool cultures often revealed only S. epidermidis. Finally, elements of "normal" flora began to appear, such as alpha streptococci in the throat and S. epidermidis in the nose and umbilicus. Few babies were colonized with group B streptococci or S. aureus. Gram-negative bacilli were frequently isolated from the nose, throat and umbilicus, not just from the stool.

Moreover, although some neonates were colonized with E. coli, a great number of babies acquired specific strains of Klebsiella, Enterobacter and Citrobacter, the antibiotic-resistant nosocomial pathogens that happened to be prevalent in the NICU at the time. Stool appeared to be the major reservoir of these gram-negative bacteria, and other sites were never colonized in the absence of stool colonization with the same strain. The risk of acquiring Klebsiella, Enterobacter and Citrobacter, particularly in the stool, increased dramatically the longer babies stayed in the NICU (Figure 3).

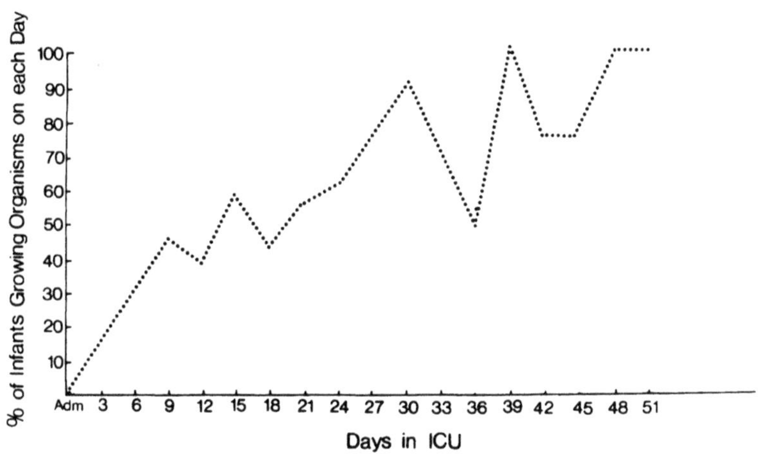

Figure 3. Stool colonization with Klebsiella, Enterobacter or Citrobacter.

By two weeks, 60 % of babies were colonized, and neonates who were unfortunate enough to require intensive care for one month had almost a 100 % chance of acquiring nosocomial organisms. Similar patterns of colonization have been noted in other nurseries, although the organisms colonizing the babies obviously differed. For example, 80 % of babies remaining in the Brown University NICU for one month developed stool colonization with a nosocomial strain of E. coli K1 (15).

It is important to recognize that nosocomially-acquired gram-negative bacilli are not just a trivial component of the neonate's stool flora. In our studies it was not uncommon to find $>10^8$ cfu of Klebsiella per gram of stool. Moreover, once babies were colonized, they tended to remain colonized. Other investigators have noted that most babies carry NICU-acquired, R-factor bearing gram-negative bacilli in the stool for a year or more (16). Therefore, when these babies are readmitted to other areas of the hospital at a later date, they may provide a reservoir for further spread of their pathogens to other children.

In the hectic, sometimes chaotic atmosphere of our old NICU, it is not hard to imagine how Klebsiella and other gram-negative bacteria which ultimately caused nosocomial infections were so quickly transferred to newly admitted babies. These new arrivals were confronted by a room full of babies who were already heavily colonized and were excreting billions of gram-negative bacilli in their copious stools. Given the under-staffing and lack of sinks in the nursery, it is not surprising that hand washing was often neglected and that organisms were carried from baby to baby on the hands of personnel. Indeed, unannounced hand cultures of the NICU staff revealed that the hands of 11 of 16 nurses and four of four physicians were heavily contaminated with the same gram-negative bacilli that had colonized the babies under their care. Of course, there is always the potential for dissemination of bacteria in the nursery due to contamination of a common vehicle such as a soap dispenser or a blood pressure transducer. However, in outbreak after outbreak of gram-negative nosocomial infection, the stools of the babies have provided the reservoir of the epidemic strain and contaminated hands have provided the means for spreading the organism throughout the nursery.

Unfortunately, the best efforts of the infection control team and nursery staff are often insufficient to prevent nosocomial acquisition of gram-negative bacilli in an intensive care setting. In an outbreak of gram-negative nosocomial infection, even vigerous measures such as cohorting of patients and nursing staff may fail to stem the inexorable spread of the epidemic strain from baby to baby. Some investigators, perhaps frustrated by the difficulty of policing handwashing by the intensive care staff, have chosen to investigate other methods for preventing colonization of neonates with gram negative bacilli. One rather novel approach has evolved from the work of Dr Katherine Sprunt's group at Babies Hospital in New York. Dr Sprunt and her colleagues have attempted to prevent colonization and infection with gram-negative bacilli by implanting strains of alpha streptococci in the pharynx of high risk neonates. This approach, which is generally called "bacterial interference", is not totally unfamiliar to physicians who were in the infection control field in the 1960's when S. aureus was the scourge of countless nurseries. In a desperate attempt to halt the epidemics of staphylococcal infection, Shinefield colonized the nose and umbilicus of babies with S. aureus phage type 502A in the hope that this allegedly benign staphylococcal strain would help neonates resist colonization and infection by more virulent phage types such as 80/81 (17). This strategy was not altogether unsuccessful, but it fell into disuse after some babies developed S. aureus 502A infection. As the staphylococcal problem began to wane at the end of the decade, the small risk of infection with 502A became unacceptable.

Dr Sprunt's curiosity in the phenomenon of bacterial interference was first stimulated when she and her colleagues noticed that cardiac surgery patients who had alpha streptococci in the pharynx rarely developed gram-negative nococomial colonization and infection. She hypothesized that the alpha streptococci were producing a substance which inhibited growth of gram-negative pathogens in the pharynx, since such inhibition could be demonstrated in vitro. Subsequently, she discovered that critically ill babies who had pharyngeal colonization with gram-negative bacilli were at very high risk for developing nosocomial infections with the colonizing strain, but that both colonization and infection were infrequent if babies had abundant growth of alpha streptococci on throat culture (18). Emboldened by these intriguing observations, she decided to deliberately implant a strain of alpha streptococci in the pharynx of high-risk babies. A strain was selected which looked particularly promising in in vitro studies; it was also moderately resistant to penicillin so that it would not be eradicted from the pharynx by the antibiotic therapy neonates were likely to receive. In her studies to date, Dr Sprunt has found that neonates who were colonized successfully with this strain of alpha streptococci appeared to have a reduced incidence of gram negative colonization and infection. In some babies who had already been colonized with gram-negative bacilli, inoculation of the alpha streptococci seemed to produce a precipitous decline in the concentration of gram-negative bacilli in the pharynx, sometimes to levels which were undetectable by culture. In further studies, Dr Sprunt's alpha streptococcus has been used in an attempt to control a small outbreak of aminoglycoside resistant gram-negative nosocomial infection at Children's Hospital in Louisville, Kentucky (4). Implantation was associated with eradication of aminoglycoside resistant bacteria from the pharynx of a few babies, although other control measures were instituted concurrently.

Dr Sprunt's work is of great interest. However, in our studies of bacterial colonization in the NICU, babies who had alpha streptococci in their pharynx did not appear to be protected from acquiring gram-negative bacilli (14) : Of the 20 patients in whom alpha streptococci could not be detected on pharyngeal culture, six (30 %) were colonized with gram-negative bacilli. On the other hand, 14 of the 36 patients (39 %) who had moderate to abundant growth of alpha strepto-cocci from two or more sequential pharyngeal cultures subsequently were colonized with gram-negative bacilli (X^2 = 0.4) and alpha streptococci and gram-negative bacilli were often isolated from the same culture. It should be noted, however, that our studies were not specifically designed to evaluate the phenomenon of bacterial interference, our definitions of "significant" colonization differed from those used by Dr Sprunt, and we do not know whether the strains of streptococci recovered from our patients would have inhibited the growth of gram-negative bacilli in vitro. Dr Sprunt's interesting observations certainly deserve further investigation.

In our laboratory, we have based our research on the premise that a successful approach to the prevention of bacterial colonization is likely to spring from an understanding of the colonization process itself.* Colonization of mucosal surfaces often involves actual adherence of bacteria to the epithelium, and this is generally the result of a specific interaction between structures on the surface of the organism (ligands) and receptors on the surface of the host epithelium. Bacteria which can adhere tightly to these surfaces may resist normal host defenses designed to sweep them away, such as the flow of secretions, peristalsis and ciliary action. Close apposition to mucosal surfaces also insures contact between the epithelium and toxins elaborated by the organism and probably facilitates microbial invasion of the epithelium.

A variety of microbial surface structures can function as ligands. For example, lipoteichoic acid mediates the attachment of group A streptococci to pharyngeal epithelium. However, in most cases the ability of bacteria to adhere to epithelial cells has been associated with protein surface structures called "pili" or "fimbriae" because of their rod or hair-like shape. Piliated bacteria appear to be critical to the pathogenesis of a number of infectious diseases, including gonorrhea, enterotoxigenic E. coli gastroenteritis and urinary tract infection, to name only a few of the most thoroughly investigated infections.

---

*The work described in this paper was performed by Nicholas, Guerina, Herbert Clegg, Woodrow Kessler, Solomon Langermann, Frank Scannapieco and Victoria Guerina in the Laboratories of the Division of Infectious Diseases, Children's Hospital Medical Center, Boston, Massachusetts.

To determine whether neonatal colonization with gram-negative bacilli involves pilus-mediated adherence to mucosal surfaces, we decided to study an organism which can cause nosocomial infections but is usually thought of as a perinatally acquired pathogen - E. coli Kl. Although there are more than 100 capsular (K) serotypes of E. coli, strains which have the Kl capsular polysaccharide (a polymer of N-acetyl neuraminic acid) are responsible for 80 % of cases of E. coli meningitis (19). Moreover, neonates with meningitis caused by E. coli Kl are more likely to have an unfavorable outcome than babies infected with other capsular serotypes. We selected E. coli Kl for study not only because of its known virulence, but also because of our familiarity with a well-studied neonatal rat model of Kl bacteremia and meningitis (20). Confirming the work of other investigators (20), we found that rats fed E. coli Kl shortly after birth experienced a high rate of bacteremia. Oral feedings of 6.0×10^6 cfu of E. coli Kl delivered atraumatically via an Eppendorf pipette produced bacteremia rates of 20-81 %, depending on the strain used. Bacteremia generally was detectable several days after oral challenge. Other E. coli serotypes, including an acapsular variant of Kl, produced negligible bacteremia. Having documented the virulence of E. coli Kl, we then investigated the time course and sites of colonization in the rat model. Streptomycin resistant mutants were used to facilitate detection of the challenge strain in cultures of the throat and intestine. Oropharyngeal cultures were obtained by vigorously swabbing the posterior pharynx of the animals and plating the swabs directly on agar containing streptomycin. Quantitative cultures of the intestine were obtained by sacrificing the animals on days one, three, five and seven after feeding. One cm. segments of duodenum, jejunum, ileum and colon, including the luminal contents, were homogenized and appropriate dilutions were plated on the selective medium. E. coli Kl promptly and reliably colonized the entire alimentary canal from oropharynx to colon. Colonization persisted for the seven days of the study, and examination of a limited number of animals revealed continued colonization until weaning. In the intestine, the concentration of bacteria in the duodenum and jejunum was relatively uniform, but increased approximately 10-fold in the ileum and about 1,000-fold in the colon. For example, the mean concentration of E. coli Kl strains (expressed as $\log_{10}$ cfu/cm ± S.D.) by seven days post-feeding was 4.0 ± 1.3 cfu/cm in the duodenum, 4.3 ± 1.3 cfu/cm in the jejunum, 5.2 ± 1.0 cfu/cm in the ileum and 7.2 ± 0.7 cfu/cm in the colon. However, if the intestinal segments were gently washed to remove their luminal contents prior to homogenization and culture, only very small number of E. coli Kl were isolated, suggesting that the bacteria were not tightly adherent to the intestinal epithelium. Preliminary results of studies using organ culture and electronmicroscopy have confirmed that E. coli are largely confined to the lumen and are not adherent to the mucosal surface of the bowel. Therefore, we have turned our attention to the oropharynx, where stable colonization with E. coli Kl was noted in more than 90 % of animals. Our primary goal has been to determine whether colonization is associated with pilus-mediated adherence to pharyngeal epithelium.

In order to have confidence in this work, it was first necessary to have control of the surface characteristics of the E. coli we were feeding to the neonatal rats. Specifically, it was critical to know the phase of piliation of the Kl challenge strain. E. coli are able to express more than one type of pilus and some of our laboratory strains of E. coli Kl can manufacture at least two major classes. Like virtually every strain of E. coli, our Kl strains have the capacity to express so-called type 1 pili, which are also aptly referred to as "common" pili. These pili are easily recognized on electronmicroscopy and are readily distinguished by their ability to hemagglutinate guinea pig red blood cells in a fashion that is completely inhibited by mannose. Their production is under the control of chromosomal genes, the position of these genes on the chromosome has been mapped and the animo acid sequence of the pili is known. Some of our K1 strains also express pili which mediate mannose-resistant hemagglutination of red cells from various species. These pili are not the same as the pili which are involved in attachment of enterotoxigenic E. coli to small bowel mucosa ; even though both types of pili mediate mannose-resistant hemagglutination, the species of red cells that can be hemagglutinated differ. Some investigators have hypothesized that the K1 pili which produce mannose-resistant hemagglutination may turn out to be virulence factors. This seems to be exceedingly unlikely since one of our K1 strains does not have these pili and yet produces higher bacteremia and mortality rates in the neonatal rat model than any of our other K1 strains.

It is important to realize that these two types of pili are independently controlled and that one, both, or neither may be expressed depending on the culture media used or other environmental conditions. Thus, if an organism has the capacity to make pili, it can exist in either a piliated phase or a non-piliated phase. We have been able to separate one of our K1 strains (C94) into three distinct phases by manipulating the culture media : (1) piliated , mannose-sensitive hemagglutination (MS+MR-) ; (2) piliated, mannose-resistant hemagglutination (MS-MR+) ; and (3) non-piliated (MS-MR-). The trained observer can readily distinguish MS+MR- colonies from MS-MR- colonies when the bacteria are grown on a minimal glucose agar. Growth on a casaminoacid-yeast extract agar encourages MS-MR+ piliation. The phase of piliation can be verified easily by slide hemagglutination. In order to be able to examine the role of K1 capsule as well as pili in bacterial adherence, we created acapsular (K1-) variants of all three phases of the E. coli C94 strain. Thus, we had the following variants of C94 available to study adherence of E. coli K1 to oropharyngeal epithelium :

K1+	K1-
MS+MR-	MS+MR-
MS-MR+	MS-MR+
MS-MR-	MS-MR-

We found that K1+ and K1- strains colonized the oropharynx of the neonatal rat equally well, suggesting that capsule is not an important determinant of adherence. Of even greater significance was our discovery that we could establish oropharyngeal colonization in nearly 100 % of animals regardless of whether we fed them MS+MR-, MS-MR+ or MS-MR- E. coli. Moreover, when animals were cultured either one or seven days after oral feeding, only MS+MR- E. coli could be recovered from pharyngeal cultures, indicating that the challenge phases reverted to the type 1 piliated phase in vivo and suggesting that type 1 pili may be intimately involved in colonization of the oropharynx. Subsequently, we have demonstrated that MS+MR- bacteria adhere to isolated neonatal rat oropharyngeal cells in large numbers (> 200 bacteria/cell), whereas MS-MR- organisms do not adhere at all. This adherence can be almost completely blocked by mannose and by purified homologous type 1 pili. Furthermore, MS+MR- E. coli adhere to oropharyngeal cells obtained from the throat of premature and full-term babies, and adherence can be inhibited in a dose-response fashion by increasing concentrations of mannose and purified pili ; MS-MR- bacteria do not adhere to human cells.

These experiments strongly suggest that adherence of E. coli K1 to human pharyngeal cells is mediated by type 1 pili. If our C94 strain of E. coli K1 were the only organism which expressed type 1 pili and colonized the pharynx, these observations would have little practical significance. However, as mentioned previously, almost all E. coli strains can express type 1 pili, as can other Enterobacteriaceae, such as Klebsiella, which are potential nosocomial pathogens (21). Thus, it is conceivable that antibody generated against type 1 pili could block adherence and colonization of the oropharynx by a broad spectrum of gram-negative bacilli. Such antibody might be delivered to the pharyngeal mucosa either by direct oral feedings to high risk neonates or via the breast milk of mothers immunized with pilus vaccine. Development of vaccine or antiserum must proceed cautiously, however, since there is antigenic heterogeneity among type 1 pili, and it is unknown whether antibody directed against the pili of one strain would block pilus-mediated adherence of other strains.

At best, these are indirect and unproven approaches to the control of nosocomial colonization and infection. In the immediate future it is likely that we will continue to rely on traditional infection control techniques in our efforts to limit transmission of nosocomial pathogens. Out studies and experiences in our new NICU suggest that a highly motivated staff working in a spacious, well-designed environment can minimize the risk of nosocomial infection for even very low birth weight, critically ill neonates.

REFERENCES

1. Eisenach, K.D., Reber, R.M., Eitzman, D.V., Baer, H. 1972. Nosocomial infections due to kanamycin-resistant, R-factor carrying enteric organisms in an intensive care nursery. Pediatrics 50 : 395.
2. Hill, H.R., Hunt, C.E., Matsen, J.M. 1974. Nosocomial colonization with Klebsiella, type 26, in a neonatal intensive care unit associated with an outbreak of sepsis, meningitis and necrotizing enterocolitis. J. Pediatr. 85 : 415.
3. Hable, K.A., Matsen, J.M., Wheeler, D.J., Hunt, C.E., Quie, P.G. 1972. Klebsiella type 33 septicemia in an infant intensive care unit. J. Pediatr. 80 : 920.
4. Cook, L.N., Davis, R.S., Stover, B.H. 1980. Outbreak of amikacin-resistant Enterobacteriaceae in an intensive care nursery. Pediatrics 65 : 264.
5. Rapkin, R.H. 1976. Pseudomonas cepacia in an intensive care nursery. Pediatrics 57 : 239.
6. Hazuka, B.T., Dajani, A.S., Talbot, K., Keen, B.M. 1977. Two outbreaks of Flavobacterium meningosepticum type E in a neonatal intensive care unit. J. Clin. Microbiol. 6 : 450.
7. Ribeiro, C.D., Davis, P., Jones, D.M. 1976. Citrobacter koseri meningitis in a special care baby unit. J. Clin. Pathol. 29 : 1094.
8. Centers for Disease Control. 1979. Nosocomial meningitis caused by Citrobacter diversus - Connecticut, Florida. Morbidity Mortality Weekly Rep. 28 : 249.
9. Mayhall, C.G., Lamb, V.A., Bitar, C.M., Miller, K.B., Furse, E.Y., Kirkpatrick, B.V., Markowitz, S.M., Veazey, J.M., Macrina, F.L. 1980. Nosocomial Klebsiella infection in a neonatal unit : identification of risk factors for gastrointestinal colonization. Infection Control 1 : 239.
10. Hemming, V.G., Overall, J.C. Jr., Britt, M.R. 1976. Nosocomial infections in a newborn intensive care unit : results of forty-one months of surveillance. N. Engl. J. Med. 294 : 1310.

11. Goldmann, D.A., Durbin, W.A. Jr., Freeman, J. 1981. Nosocomial infections in a neonatal intensive care unit. J. Infect. Dis. 144 : 449.
12. Outline for surveillance and control of nosocomial infections. 1972. Centers for Disease Control, Atlanta, Ga.
13. Standards and recommendations for hospital care of newborn infants. 1977. 6th ed. Committee on Fetus and Newborn, American Academy of Pediatrics, Evanston, Ill., 25.
14. Goldmann, D.A., Leclair, J., Macone, A. 1978. Bacterial colonization of neonates admitted to an intensive care environment. J. Pediatr. 2 : 288.
15. Peter, G., Nelson, J.S. 1978. Factors affecting neonatal E. coli Kl rectal colonization. J. Pediatr. 93 : 866.
16. Damato, J.J., Eitzman, D.V., Baer, H. 1974. Persistence and dissemination in the community of R-factors of nosocomial origin. J. Infect. Dis. 129 : 205.
17. Shinefield, H.R., Ribble, J.C., Boris, M. 1971. Bacterial interference between strains of Staphylococcus aureus. 1960-1970. Am. J. Dis. Child. 121 : 148.
18. Sprunt, K., Leidy, G., Redman, W. 1978. Abnormal colonization of neonates in an intensive care unit : means of identifying neonates at risk of infection. Ped. Res. 12 : 998.
19. Glode, M.P., Sutton, A., Robbins, J.B., et al. 1977. Neonatal meningitis due to Escherichia coli Kl. J. Infect. Dis. 136 : 593.
20. Glode, M.P., Sutton, A., Moxon, E.R., Robbins, J.G. 1977. Pathogenesis of neonatal Escherichia coli meningitis : induction of bacteremia and meningitis in infant rats fed E. coli Kl. Infect. Immun. 16 : 75.
21. Duguid, J.P. 1959. Fibriae and adhesive properties in Klebsiella strains. J. Gen. Microbiol. 21 : 271.

NOSOCOMIAL INFECTIONS IN THE NEONATAL INTENSIVE CARE UNIT

J.J. ROORD, R.Ch. SENDERS, and A. FLEER*

During recent years remarkable advances have been made in the medical care of severely ill newborn infants. Regional intensive care units have been established in places throughout the world, which has reduced both morbidity and mortality in the high-risk population. With increasing obstetrical and pediatric knowledge and facilities and an increasing number of pathological pregnancies resulting in delivery of living but often severely premature infants, the mean gestational age of newborns admitted to neonatal intensive care units has decreased.

Surveys in general and pediatric hospitals have shown that intensive-care patients run a high risk of acquiring a nosocomial infection. Prematurely born neonates in a neonatal intensive care unit (NICU) may be at the greatest risk with respect to hospital infections, which not only prolong hospital stay but also contribute to life-long morbidity and to mortality. Intensive care for neonates frequently includes extensive instrumentation procedures (intubation, indwelling arterial catheters, prolonged fluid administration via peripheral veins), and frequent blood sampling is performed for diagnostic, therapeutic, and monitoring purposes.

Neonatal host defence factors

In many respects the newborn in an NICU exemplifies an immunocompromised host. Each component of the host defense is relatively immature in the newborn, and especially of the premature infant (1). In the term infant the serum level of trans-

* Laboratory for Microbiology, University of Utrecht, Utrecht, The Netherlands

placentally acquired IgG is 110% of the maternal serum level, but in premature infants the serum IgG levels are much lower. Both in vitro and in vivo, the neonatal B cells are only capable of transforming into IgM-secreting plasma cells and are unable to transform into IgG- and IgA-secreting plasma cells.

Cellular immunity too is immature. T helper cell function in newborns is diminished and T suppressor cell activity is augmented. Neonatal T cells show a good proliferative response in vitro, but decreased cytotoxic activity of neonatal T cells is a consistent finding. Cutaneous hypersensitivity is diminished. The mononuclear phagocytes (monocytes/macrophages) and granulocytes can phagocytose well, but show reduced chemotaxis, which possibly contributes to the diminished cutaneous delayed hypersensitivity. The monocytes may show a reduced efficiency in antigen processing. Complement activity is only half that found in older children and adults. The alternative pathway of complement is compromised more often than the classical pathway. Maternal factors such as malnutrition, infection, prolonged labour, placental insufficiency, and the use of such drugs as steroids, are associated with increased risk of neonatal infection.

Nursing of a neonate in an NICU may interfere with the development of a normal bacterial flora and may influence the development of a normal colonization resistance (2).

Measures for infection control

Effective control of infection in an NICU starts with the architectural design of the unit. The amount of floor space allotted for each patient must be sufficient to permit adequate performance of necessary techniques (3). Medical care for sick neonates is not provided by dwarfs!

The ventilation of the unit must provide for 10 to 15 exchanges of air per hour via high-efficiency particulate air-filters, and the air channels must not interconnect with other channels between entry and exit. A sink must be located in the immediate vicinity of each incubator. Entry into an NICU must be restricted to essential personnel and close relatives. Anyone entering the NICU should be required to wash hands and scrub to the elbow with chlorhexidine gluconate.

The floor of the unit must be cleaned daily with a damp cloth, after daily dusting of shelves, light fixtures, and so forth. Personnel with symptoms or signs of any infectious disease should be refused entry to the unit. Contact with patients should be limited to the smallest number of persons possible, and hands should be washed before and after patient contact. Disposable equipment should be used whenever possible. Monitors, pumps, isolettes, laryngoscopes, and so forth, should be cleaned and disinfected after use, and all surgical instruments and all re-usable equipment should be cleaned and sterilized after use.

Irrigation of sinks several times a day is necessary to prevent colonization with Gram-negative organisms. In 1973, the incidence in our NICU of nosocomial infection with Pseudomonas aeruginosa was 14.1%! Pseudomonas aeruginosa was isolated from many sources in the NICU: the floor, furniture, wash stands (taps and sinks), suction equipment, respiratory apparatus, hands and clothes of nurses, and the ointment used for the babies' lips. Infection from these sources was eliminated by the maintenance of rigid disinfection procedures during the following years, and this was accompanied by an enormous decrease in hospital infections due to Pseudomonas aeruginosa (14.1% in 1973, 4.9% in 1977, 2.6% in 1980). Indwelling vascular catheters, and even scalp-vein needles, constitute a major potential source of hospital infection; they should be replaced after being in situ for 48 hours.

Continuing periodic surveillance with respect to bacterial colonization has been accepted in many centres as a part of NICU routine. Infections might tend to occur especially in infants with abnormal pharyngeal colonization, and the infecting organism might be identical with the colonizing organism (4).

In a one-year survey performed in our hospital in 1977, 55 out of 181 newborns admitted to the NICU developed a nosocomial infection (5). These infections included septicaemia (15 cases), pneumonia (25 cases), and soft-tissue infections (19 cases). The most important organisms isolated from these patients were

Staphylococcus aureus (18 cases), coagulase-negative cocci (18 cases), Escherichia coli (11 cases), Pseudomonas aeruginosa (9 cases), and Klebsiella penumonia (5 cases). Four children died of the infection, all caused by Pseudomonas aeruginosa. There was an obvious positive correlation between the duration of instrumentation procedures (mechanical ventilation, arterial and venous catheters) and the occurrence of an infection.

Special precautions should be taken in the preparation of infusion fluids. In the last few years we have been confronted with an increasing frequency of bacteraemia due to Staphylococcus epidermidis. In 1981, 40 septic episodes occurred in 35 out of 275 admitted newborns: 30 of these episodes were caused by Staphylococcus epidermidis and 10 by other micro-organisms (Klebsiella spp. 1, Streptococcus faecalis 3, Staphylococcus aureus 1, enterobacter 2, Escherichia coli 2, and Bacillus cereus 1). The Staphylococcus epidermidis strains were multiple-resistant, the antibodies including penicillin, cloxacillin, and gentamicin. The infants were usually fed intravenously, and almost all of them were on antibiotic treatment. They were not seriously sick, and treatment with cephalotin was invariably successful.

Further prospective studies showed that in a period of two months, no less than 17.9% of all intravenous feeding fluids were contaminated with Staphylococcus epidermidis. Most of the cases of bacteremia occurred in infants receiving contaminated feeding fluids; 75 out of 418 batches of intravenous feeding fluid proved to be contaminated. Six times, on clinical grounds, blood of patients who had received one of these contaminated feeding fluids was cultured; all of the cultures were positive for Staphylococcus epidermidis. During 69 episodes of contaminated-fluid infusion, there were no clinical signs indicating the need for blood cultures. Host defense factors seemed to play a role in the outcome of infusion with contaminated fluids. Most of the infants were severely premature and had a very low birth weight (less than 28 weeks of gestation in 5 cases, 28 to 32 weeks in 9 cases, 32 to 36 weeks in 9, and 36 to 42 weeks in 4; 5 weighed less than 1000 gram, 7 weighed 1000 to 1500 gram, 8 weighed 1500 to 2000 gram, and 7 more than 2000 gram). In the patients who received the 343 sterile feeding fluids, only two blood samples were taken for culture on clinical grounds and both were positive.

Intravenous fluids were prepared in syringes from sterile, commercially available bottles containing glucose, electrolytes, intralipids, or amino acids. The only break in sterility we could detect was the drawing into the syringe of a small amount of NICU air, which was subsequently injected into the bottles to facilitate the drawing of fluid from the bottles into the syringe. The ward air proved to be contaminated with Staphylococcus epidermidis. Intravenous feeding fluids are now prepared in a laminar flow cabinet, but we do not yet have sufficient data to analyse the effect on hospital infections.

Enhancement of the neonatal host defense

It would seem advantageous to increase the neonatal host defence at several points in newborns at risk. For example, intravenous immunoglobulin G substitution might be useful in life-threatening neonatal infections (6); the protective, preventive effect in preterm infants is not well documented. Studies on artificially induced "normal" pharyngeal colonization by implanting α-haemolitic streptococci in the nasopharynx of high-risk newborns showed that colonization with nosocomial pathogens could be reduced significantly (2).

The mechanisms underlying the immunity provided by breast feeding have been the subject of many studies. Human milk contains, among others IgA antibodies (against a variety of enterobacteriaceae, viruses, and food proteins), macrophages, granulocytes, and B and T lymphocytes (7). Their biological significance is difficult to assess in the NICU, but after the introduction of feeding with fresh human milk we observed a significant decrease in the incidence of necrotising enterocolitis.

REFERENCES

1. Stiehm, E.M. 1980. The human neonate as an immunocompromised host. In: Infections in the immunocompromised host. Eds P.K. Peterson and P.G. Quie. Elsevier North Holland. Amsterdam. 77.
2. Goldmann, D.A. 1981. Bacterial colonization and infection in the neonate. Am. J. Med. 70: 417.
3. Goldmann, D.A., Durbin, W.A., Freeman, J. 1981. Nosocomial infections in a neonatal intensive care unit. J. Infect. Dis. 144: 449.
4. Sprunt, K., Leidy, G., Redman, W. 1978. Abnormal colonization of neonates in an intensive care unit. Pediatr. Res. 12: 998.
5. Hoogkamp-Korstanje, J.A.A., Cats, B., Senders, R.Ch., Ertbruggen van, I. 1982. Analysis of bacterial infections in a neonatal intensive care unit. J. Hosp. Infect. in press.
6. Muralt, G., Sidiropoulos, D. 1981. Intravenous Ig-substitution therapy in the treatment of septicemia in preterm neonates. In: Immunohemotherapy. Ed. U.E. Nydegger. Academic Press. London, New York, Toronto, Sydney, San Francisco. 313.
7. Freier, S., Eidelman, A.I., eds. 1980. Human milk. Excerpta Medica. Amsterdam.

DISCUSSION EDITED BY J.J. ROORD

Rubin: I would like to mention the role of the piliated strains of E. coli in urinary tract infections. Increasing attention has been given to P fimbrae, which have a substance that cross-reacts with the bloodgroup P substance. In Sweden, Catharine Svanborg Eden recently showed that these P fimbrae are present in 90% of the pyelonephritis versus less than 20% of the strains causing cystitis or just colonizing the lower urogenital tract. The question can be posed whether these P fimbrae are of importance in colonization of the gastro-intestinal tract.

Goldmann: The original studies in the urinary tract showed that there was an adherence to the mucus of the genito-urniary tract and not to the epithelial cells. Under the conditions used for the study of mannose-resistant pili, they seemed to be the kind of pili that Dr. Svenborg Eden described. No role could be found for these pili in the ileum or oropharynx.

van der Meer: I would like to point to the different colonization patterns observed in the gut of breast-fed and formula-fed children. Have any attempts been made to colonize the children with lactobacilli? Do you have any information about colonization with anaerobes in these infants?

Goldmann: We have looked for an effect of breast milk, but because of bad banking of breast milk, none of the babies has been able to make a reasonable attempt at breast feeding. It would certainly be worthwhile to investigate the effect of fresh human milk. Information concerning the anaerobes is available, but not from our own work. The critically ill neonate rapidly develops an anaerobic pattern similar to that of the adult. Intensive-care babies acquire Bacteroides fragilis, Clostridium perfringens, and so on.

van den Broek:How do you explain the differences in the frequency with which Klebsiella is involved in the nosocomial infections in Boston. In Boston this was a major pathogen whereas in Utrecht Klebsiella was only of minor importance.

Goldmann: I think that Klebsiella in the nursery is primarily a pathogen acquired from nurses. It seems to be a nosocomially spread strain in the neonatal intensive care unit, because of the antibiotic resistance patterns in the biotyping and even of the serum types. I cannot offer a good explanation.

van Furth: Is there a specific policy for antibiotic administration in Boston and in Utrecht?

Goldmann: We are a referral hospital and so we have no specific policy on immediate post-partum antibiotics. If a baby has had a very premature rupture of the membranes, particularly if the mother has a fever or foul amniotic fluid, that baby will be given antibiotics. In the very low birthweight infants, the signs of infection are so non-specific that more than 80% of the babies were given antibiotics within the first ten days. So for all practical purposes, the great majority end up receiving something.

Roord: If there is just a little non-specific sign of infection the child will be given antibiotics. Utrecht too is a referral hospital, so 70% of the newborns had had antibotics before admission. Usually penicillin/gentamicin or ampicillin/gentamicin is given; in cases of a hospital-acquired infection, cephalotin/ gentamicin is often used because of Staphylococcus epidermidis, but the clinical data determine the final choice.

Goldmann: We have the same policy, but we also culture for gentamicin-resistant micro-organisms. If any gentamicin-resistant micro-organism is detected in the nursery, the policy is to give ampicillin/amikacin. Moxalactam is very popular now because of its broad spectrum and good penetration of the CSF. The combination of penicillin and moxalactam becomes a regimen of choice in cases of meningitis.

Roord: The difference between the numbers of nosocomial infections in Boston and Utrecht is remarkable, and I wonder what the explanation might be. One-fourth of the newborns in Utrecht had an infection on admission.

Goldmann: I cannot recall the exact percentage of infected newborns on admission, but I think would be less than 5%. The most important diagnosis by far was the respiratory distress syndrome. About once a month a baby is admitted for cross-infection.

Hoogkamp-Korstanje: We have identified the Gram-positive staphylococci as micrococci of certain groups and Staphylococcus saphrophyticus; 40% of the children were colonized with these strains, and these strains were multiple-resistant including to penicillin, methicillin, and cloxacillin.

Goldmann: Up to 1977, we called those cocci "Staphylococcus non-aureus". Subsequently, they were identified on the basis of neomycin resistance, but what we were seeing was Staphylococcus epidermidis. The saphrophyticus strains are quite susceptible to the betalactam antibiotics and most of the Staphylococcus epidermidis strains are resistant to aminoglycosides and other antibiotics as well.

INFECTION IN THE RENAL TRANSPLANT PATIENT

NINA E. TOLKOFF-RUBIN and R.H. RUBIN

Over the past two decades, remarkable progress has been made in dealing with the twin barriers to successful renal transplantation-rejection and infection. Twenty years ago, more than 50 % of transplanted patients were dying of infection in the first year post-transplant, and the kidneys in less than half of the remaining patients continued to function. Today, at the best transplant centers, the one-year patient survival rate for recipients of kidneys from living related donors is >95 % and for recipients of kidneys from cadaveric donors >90 %, with graft survival rates of >85 % and >65 %, respectively. Advances in the use of immunosuppression, in surgical techniques, and in the prevention and treatment of infection have all contributed to these improved results. It must be emphasized, however, that more than 80 % of transplant recipients still develop significant infection, with 26 % of them dying as a direct result, and much has yet to be accomplished in terms of preventing and treating such infections (1, 2). Our purpose here is to outline a practical approach for achieving this objective.

MANAGEMENT OF IMMUNOSUPPRESSIVE THERAPY

Perhaps the greatest lesson to come out of the early transplant experience was that there was a limit to the amount of corticosteroid a patient could safely tolerate. In contrast, azathioprine, the other established component of most immunosuppressive regimens is relatively well tolerated as long as the dosage administered (usually 75-150 mg/day) does not result in undue bone marrow suppression, with peripheral granulocyte counts being maintained at levels $>2500/mm^3$ and platelet counts >100,000/mm^3. A great effort has been made to decrease the amount of immunosuppression required by means of more optimal tissue typing and matching of donor organ to potential recipient, with DR matching being the most exciting new developement in this area. In addition, recipients are better prepared for transplantation, with pre-transplant transfusion playng a significant role in decreasing the incidence and severity of allograft rejection. By decreasing the extent of rejection, advances in both of these areas have decreased the amount of immunosuppression required to keep a functioning graft in place, and thereby decreased the risk of infection (1, 2).

In the past, it was fashionable to attribute infection to one or another component of the immunosuppressive regimen. It has now become apparent that much more important is the net state of immunosuppression produced, with steroids, azathioprine, antithymocyte globulin (ATG), uremia, viral infections, etc., all contributing to the patient's immunosuppressed state. For example, we have shown that when ATG is added to a full program of prednisone and azathioprine the incidence of cytomegalovirus (CMV) viremia and clinical syndromes due to this virus are significantly increased, and that the beneficial effects of prophylactic interferon are attenuated. If, however, the same dose of ATG is combined with an immunosuppressive program in which the prednisone and azathioprine dosage is halved, then the excess morbidity and potential mortality engendered by this virus are eliminated, without decreasing the antirejection effects of the combined program (3).

Perhaps the most exciting development in the management of immunosuppression that should result in a decrease in both allograft rejection and complicating infection is the monitoring of the level of T-lymphocyte subpopulations in the circulation. It has been shown that particular T-lymphocyte subsets, namely the helper-inducer and suppressor-cytotoxic cell populations, play important regulatory roles in the immune response. Such immunoregulatory T-cell subsets can be demonstrated not only by functional assays, but also by the use of specific antibodies to surface antigens that are different for each of these populations of cells. In particular, the use of the mococlonal antibodies OKT3 (all T-lymphocytes), OKT4 (helper-inducer lymphocytes) and OKT8 (suppressor-cytotoxic lymphocytes), when coupled with flow cytometry techniques, permits the rapid quantitation of the immunoregulatory T-cell populations. Using these techniques in renal transplant patients, it has been shown that a normal to increased ratio of helper to suppressor-cytotoxic cells (a ratio $\geq$1.2) is associated with rejection, while a decreased ratio is associated with cytomegalovirus and/or EB virus infection, and, possibly, an increased risk of opportunistic superinfection. Such data may permit more precise management of immunosuppressive therapy in the individual patient instead of relying on the standard protocols that have been employed in the past (4, 5).

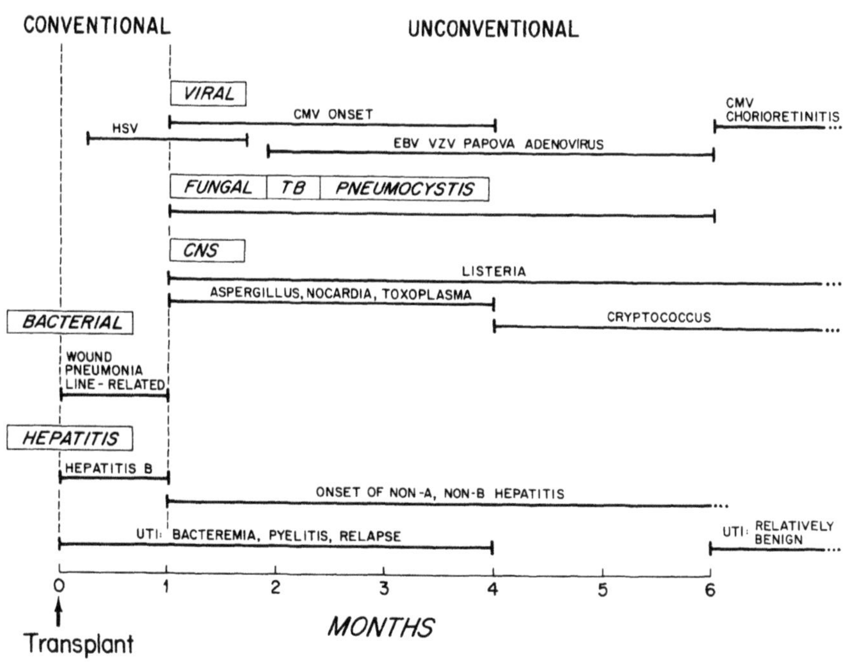

FIGURE 1. Timetable of infection in the renal transplant patient. Reprinted by permission of the American Journal of Medicine from Rubin, et al (2).

It is now apparent that there is a predictable timetable for the occurrence of specific infections in the renal transplant patient (Fig. 1). There are three separate time periods, with different types of infection being expected during each : the first month post-transplant, the period 1 to 6 months post-transplant, and the period more than six months post-transplant. In the first month post-transplant, opportunistic (protozan, fungal, and nocardial) infections are almost nonexistent, unless a major nosocomial hazard is present. Instead, the major causes of infection are the residuals of pre-transplant difficulties (i.e., hepatitis acquired on dialysis), or the bacterial wound, pulmonary, urinary tract, or intravenous line-related infections seen in any postoperative patient. The effects of such infections, however, tend to be much greater in these immunosuppressed patients (1, 2).

The time period 1 to 6 months post-transplant is the period during which the incidence of infection, particularly life-threatening opportunistic infection, is highest. This is due to two factors : the cumulative effects of immunosuppression have taken effect, and cytomegalovirus infection, which itself has important immunosuppressing effect, is occurring. Thus, the clinician must be particularly alert for the occurrence of infection in this period, as successful management of opportunistic infection is predicated upon early diagnosis and agressive therapy (1, 2).

In the late post-transplant period (>6 months post-transplant) three patterns of infection are observed : those patients who have done well and are now on minimal immunosuppression with good renal function tend to get only those infections that are present in the general community, i.e., influenza, urinary tract infection, or pneumococcal pneumonia ; those patients who acquired viral infection earlier in their post-transplant course may have chronic effects from these, with the best examples of this phenomenon being chronic active hepatitis and cytomegalovirus chorioretinitis ; and those patients with chronic rejection (serum creatinines > 2 mg/dl) on higher levels of immunosuppression who remain at risk for opportunistic infection, particularly that due to Cryptococcus neoformans and Listeria monocytogenes (1, 2).

This timetable of the occurrence of infection in the renal transplant patient can be useful in two ways. First, it serves as a guide in diagnosing the transplant patient who presents with fever, pneumonia, or other clinical syndromes possibly due to infection at different times post-transplant. Second, it can be an important clue to unusual epidemiologic hazards. Exceptions to this timetable suggest unusual and potentially correctable exposures. In particular, any transplant recipient with an opportunistic infection in the first month post-transplant should trigger a search for an unusual nosocomial hazard. In recent years, epidemics of invasive aspergillosis due to Aspergillus spores contaminating weatherproofing and fireproofing materials, of Legionnaires' disease due to contamination of a variety of water sources within the hospital, and of Legionella micdadei infection (the Pittsburgh Pneumonia Agent) among renal transplant patients due to nosocomial exposure emphasize the importance of this concept (1, 2).

INFECTION OF PARTICULAR IMPORTANCE IN THE RENAL TRANSPLANT PATIENT

Wound infection

Infections of the transplant wound have traditionally been regarded as a major problem in renal transplantation, occurring in as many as 56 % of patients, with 75 % of deep peri-allograft infections resulting in allograft removal and many lives being lost due to systemic sepsis arising from this site or massive hemorrhage due to infection at the vascular anastomosis (6). That such events are not inevitable is suggested by the experience at the University of Minnesota. This group has reported an overall incidence among 439 consecutive transplants of 6.1 %. If, however, those secondary to hematoma or urinary fistula are excluded, then the incidence of wound infection is only 1.6 %, with all of these being superficial infections (7). Although some transplant groups have placed great emphasis upon the efficacy of prophylactic antibiotics in preventing wound infections (8), we have observed an infection rate in primary wounds of < 2 % without the use of systemic antimicrobial prophylaxis. We feel that this experience, coupled with the Minnesota observations, indicates that the most important factor in preventing wound sepsis is not antibiotics, but rather the technical quality of the surgery performed (2).

Cytomegalovirus infection

By far the most common and probably most important infection occurring in transplant patients is that due to cytomegalovirus (CMV). CMV is ubiquitous among renal transplant recipients, with 60 to 96 % of these individuals having clinical and/or laboratory evidence of the infection post-transplant - with virtually all having their onset 1 to 4 months post-transplant. The known clinical effects of CMV can be grouped into three categories : (1) the production of a variety of infectious disease syndromes by itself (i.e., fever, pneumonia, chorioretinitis, leukopenia, thrombocytopenia, hepatitis, and, possibly, gastrointestinal tract ulcerations); (2) the production of a severe depression in host defenses that is over and above that caused by immunosuppressive therapy and that predisposes to superinfection with such agents as Aspergillus species, Pneumocystis carinii, and Listeria monocytogenes ; (3) the probable production of allograft injury manifested as a glomerulopathy distinct from classical rejection which is unresponsive to usual immunosuppressive therapy. It is these last two CMV effects that appear to be clinically most important in the renal transplant patient (1, 2).

Epidemiologically, two patterns of CMV disease are recognized : (1) primary CMV disease in which the transplant recipient is sero-negative prior to transplant and receives the virus within latently infected kidney allografts or leukocyte-containing blood transfusions from sero-positive donors ; and (2) reactivation CMV disease in which sero-positive allograft recipients reactivate their own latent infection post-transplant. In both instances, the immunosuppressive therapy administered and the rejection processes that follow placement of an allograft appear to activate latent virus and make it clinically manifest. Currently published data would suggest that approximately 2/3 of patients at risk for primary disease develop symptomatic CMV, while less than 1/3 of those at risk for reactivation disease do. Overall, however, since at many transplant centers 60 to 90 % of the patients who receive transplants are sero-positive pre-transplant, reactivation disease has an effect that is at least equal to that of primary disease on the outcome of clinical renal transplantation (1, 2).

Clinical management of CMV infection thus far has been unsatisfactory, with no specific therapy yet available. Prophylaxis with human leukocyte interferon and an attenuated CMV vaccine appear promising, but are as yet only experimental. Therefore, emphasis at present must be placed on decreasing immunosuppression (perhaps guided by the reversed helper/suppressor ratio seen in these patients) and having a low threshold for placing the patients on trimethoprim-sulfamethoxazole prophylaxis/therapy because of the particularly close association between CMV and Pneumocystis carinii (1).

Other viruses

At present there is clear-cut evidence that the herpes group viruses (CMV, EB virus, varicella-zoster virus, and herpes simplex virus), a variety of hepatitis viruses, and, possibly adenoviruses and papovaviruses have a significant impact on renal transplant patients. Although space does not permit a detailed review of each of these agents, several points are worthy of comment here :

EB virus probably produces infectious disease syndromes similar to those described for CMV - both by itself and in predisposing to superinfection (it, too, produces a reversal in the normal helper/suppressor-cytotoxic cell ratio). Even more interesting is the increasing evidence that EB virus is closely linked to the pathogenesis of an unusual lymphoproliferative syndrome observed in transplant patients, particularly those treated with such experimental immunosuppressive agents as cyclosporin A (1, 2, 9). One such patient has been described whose lymphoproliferative disease initially responded to anti-EB virus chemotherapy (with acyclovir, an agent with little if any conventional anti-lymphoma effect) (10).

Dermatomal varicella-zoster virus infection due to reactivation of latent virus occurs in 7 to 9 % of renal transplant recipients, is usually self-limited, and rarely disseminates. In contrast to the rather benign course of zoster in this population, primary varicella infection can be quite virulent. Therefore, renal transplant patients (particularly children) without previous history of varicella who have a significant exposure to the virus should be strongly considered for zoster immune globulin prophylaxis (1, 2).

Localized herpes simplex infection, both oral and anogenital, occurs commonly in the first month post-transplant. Such localized disease may be quite severe, and in the case of oral-labial disease, may lead to aspiration or inadequate nutrition. Every effort should be made in patients with oral lesions to avoid nasogastric tubes or endotracheal intubation, as such mucosal trauma can lead to severe herpetic esophagitis and/or tracheitis. Fortunately, disseminated herpes simplex infection is quite rare in this population (1, 2, 11).

Abnormalities of liver function tests are quite common in this patient population, with some 6 to 16 % of patients developing chronic hepatitis. Although in the past hepatitis B was the major cause of this problem, so-called non-A, non-B hepatitis now accounts for more than 2/3 of such cases. This infection, too, appears to have immunosuppressing effects, as indicated by a high risk of extra-hepatic infection on the one hand and a increased rate of allograft survival on the other. This increase in graft survival is more than compensated for by a mortality rate, predominantly from extra-hepatic sepsis, more than twice as high as in the non-hepatitis patients (12, 13).

Papovaviruses are receiving increasing attention in this population, as the causative agents of progressive multifocal leukoencephalopathy, and as possible causative agents of ureteral stenosis and the development of such long-term complications as post-transplant diabetes, arteriosclerosis, and malignancy (1, 2, 11, 14).

Adenoviruses, both conventional ones and newly discovered types (adenoviruses 34 and 35) as yet only found in this patient population, appear to cause both respiratory tract and urinary tract infection in renal transplant recipients at a rate greater than that observed in the general population (1, 2, 11).

Urinary tract infection

Infection of the urinary tract (UTI) has been reported to occur in some 35 to 79 % of renal transplant recipients, with different impacts depending upon the time post-transplant when it occurs. UTI presenting in the first three months post-transplant is frequently associated with overt pyelonephritis, bacteremia, allograft dysfunction, and a high rate of relapse when treated with a conventional 10-day course of antibiotics (but which responds well to a 6-week course of therapy). Recently, a randomized study has shown that the administration of one double-strength tablet of trimethoprim-sulfamethoxazole per day for the first four months post-transplant is quite effective in preventing UTI, with virtual eradication of gram-negative sepsis of urinary tract origin (1, 2).

UTI, beginning later in the post-transplant course, if uncomplicated by anatomical abnormalities, is usually benign, can be managed with a conventional 10-14 day course of antibiotics, is rarely associated with a bacteremia or requires hospitalization, and has an excellent prognosis (1, 2).

One special form of UTI that merits attention in this population is that due to Candida species. Such infection, even if asymptomatic, can result in obstructing fungal balls at the ureterovesical junction, with deterioration of renal function and possible systemic dissemination from this site.

Bacteremia

The major source of bacteremia in the renal transplant patient has always been the urinary tract, with 60 to 70 % of bacteremias coming from this source (15). However, with better surgical technique (so that the incidence of ureteral anastomotic complications is now <5 %), agressive treatment of those infections that occur (i.e., for six weeks if occurring in the first three months post-transplant), and with trimethoprim-sulfamethoxazole prophylaxis, gram-negative sepsis of urinary tract origin has virtually disappeared. We ourselves have not had a case among the last 100 renal transplant patients cared for at our institution. The two major causes of bacteremia at our institution are Listeria monocytogenes and intravenous line-related bacteremia (particularly due to staphylococcal species). It is not that these have increased in frequency. It is just that other causes of bacteremia have been controlled (1, 2).

Pneumonia

A number of extensive reviews of pulmonary infection in the renal transplant recipient and other immunosuppressed populations have been published recently (1, 2, 16), as this is the most frequent cause of infectious disease mortality in this patient population. For example, at the Massachusetts General Hospital between 1966 and 1978, 54 of 227 renal transplant recipients (24 %) presented with fever and pulmonary infiltrates. In 27 of the 54 episodes (50 %) the pulmonary process contributed directly to the death of the patient and those accounted for 50 % of the deaths observed in the entire renal transplant patient population. Although primary pulmonary infection responded well to therapy when diagnosed early, superinfection continues to be an unsolved problem, causing virtually all of these deaths.

The etiologies of pneumonia in this population are well outlined in Fig. 1 - conventional bacterial infection in the first month post-transplant, CMV and/or opportunistic infection in the middle period, and either opportunistic or conventional viral and bacterial infection in the late period (depending on the level of immunosuppression and degree of chronic rejection present, as previously described). It has been clearly demonstrated that an agressive diagnostic approach involving trans-tracheal aspiration, percutaneous lung biopsy or fiberoptic bronchoscopy with transbronchial biopsy, or, even, open lung biopsy will be rewarded with a high rate of patient salvage (1, 2, 16).

Central nervous system infection

Between 5 and 10 % of renal transplant patients develop infection of the central nervous system (CNS) post-transplant. Four patterns of clinical disease may be observed :
(1) acute meningitis, which is almost invariably due to Listeria monocytogenes ; (2) a subacute-chronic meningitis, which is usually due to Cryptococcus neoformans (although in endemic areas Mycobacterium tuberculosis or Coccidioides immitis can present in a similar fashion) ; (3) focal brain infection, occasionally due to Listeria monocytogenes, Toxoplasma gendii, or Nocardia asteroides, but most commonly to Aspergillus infection metastatic from a site of active pulmonary infection ; (4) a progressive dementia, due to progressive multifocal leukoencephalopathy. Perhaps the most important point to be remembered by the clinician dealing with such immunosuppressed patients as renal transplant recipients is that the clinical presentation may be insidious - without meningismus or coma until very late in the clinical course. The major indication for a CNS evaluation for infection in this patient population is the presence of an unexplained headache, particularly if the headache is accompanied by fever (17).

CONCLUSION

The incidence of infection in the renal transplant patient is directly related to the net immunosuppressive effect achieved and the duration of time over which this therapy is administered. Recognition of these facts has led to the construction of an expected timetable for when in the post-transplant course each infection should occur. Exceptions to this timetable suggest either excess nosocomial hazard, particularly if opportunistic infection are involved, or that the problem was present, albeit unrecognized, prior to transplantation.

Much has been accomplished over the last two decades in overcoming the effects of the twin barriers to successful transplantation - rejection and infection. For the most part, bacterial infections have come under control. The challenge for the future is to develop better means of preventing and treating viral infection, particularly CMV and EB virus, protecting patients against nosocomial infection, and designing more specific immunosuppressive therapy. Promising leads are now available for achieving these goals.

From the Dialysis-transplantation and Infectious Disease Units of the Medical Service of the Massachusetts General Hospital and the Department of Medicine, Harvard Medical School, Boston, Massachusetts, U.S.A.

REFERENCES

1. Rubin, R.H. 1981. Infection in the renal transplant patient. In R.H. Rubin and L.S. Young (eds.). Clinical approach to infection in the compromised host. Plenum Publishing Corp., New York, 553.
2. Rubin, R.H., Wolfson, J.S., Cosimi, A.B., Tolkoff-Rubin, N.E. 1981. Infection in the renal transplant recipient. Am. J. Med. 70 : 405.
3. Rubin, R.H., Cosimi, A.B., Hirsch, M.S., et al. 1981. Effects of anti-thymocyte globulin on cytomegalovirus infection in renal transplant recipients. Transplantation. 31 : 143.
4. Cosimi, A.B., Colvin, R.B., Burton, R.C., et al. 1981. Use of monoclonal antibodies to T-cell subsets for immunologic monitoring and treatment in recipients of renal allografts. N. Engl. J. Med. 305 : 308.
5. Rubin, R.H., Carney, W.P., Schooley, R.T., et al. 1981. The effect of infection on T-lymphocyte subpopulations : a preliminary report. Int. J. Immunopharmacol. 3 : 307.

6. Lee, H.M., Madge, G.E., Mendez-Picon, G., et al. 1978. Surgical complications in renal transplant recipients. Surg. Clin. North Am. 58 : 285.
7. Kyriakides, G.K., Simmons, R.L., Najarian, J.S. 1975. Wound infections in renal transplant wounds : pathogenetic and prognostic factors. Ann. Surg. 186 : 770.
8. Tilney, N.L., Strom, T.B., Vineyard, G.C., et al. 1978. Factors contributing to the declining mortality rate in renal transplantation. N. Engl. J. Med. 229 : 1321.
9. Marker, S.C., Ascher, N.L., Kalis, J.M., et al. 1979. Epstein-Barr virus antibody responses and clinical illness in renal transplant recipients. Surgery. 85 : 433.
10. Hanto, D.W., Frizzera, G., Gajl-Peczalska, K.J. 1982. Epstein-Barr virus induced B-cell lymphoma after renal transplantation, acyclovir therapy and transition from a polyclonal to monoclonal B-cell proliferation. N. Engl. J. Med. (in press).
11. Ho, M. 1977. Virus infections after transplantation in man ; brief review. Arch. Virol. 55 : 1.
12. Ware, A.J., Luby, J.P., Hollinger, B., et al. 1979. Etiology of liver disease in renal transplant patients. Ann. Intern. Med. 91 : 364.
13. LaQuaglia, M.P., Tolkoff-Rubin, N.E., Dienstag, J.L., et al. 1981. Impact of hepatitis on renal transplantation. Transplantation. 32 : 504.
14. Hogan, T.F., Borden, E.C., McBain, J.A., et al. 1980. Human polyomavirus infections with JC virus and BK virus in renal transplant patients. Ann. Intern. Med. 92 : 373.
15. Myerowitz, R.L., Medeiros, A.A., O'Brien, T.F. 1972. Bacterial infection in renal homotransplant recipients ; a study of fifty three bacteremic episodes. Am. J. Med. 53 : 308.
16. Ramsey, P.G., Rubin, R.H., Tolkoff-Rubin, N.E., et al. 1980. The renal transplant patient with fever and pulmonary infiltrates ; etiology, clinical manifestations and management. Medicine. 59 : 206.
17. Hooper, D., Pruitt, A.A., Rubin, R.H. 1982. Infections of the central nervous system in the immunocompromised host. Medicine 61 : 166.

FACTORS CONTRIBUTING TO AN INCREASED INFECTION RATE AFTER KIDNEY TRANSPLANTATION

J.P. VAN HOOFF and P.J. VAN DEN BROEK

INTRODUCTION

The dosages of corticosteroids applied after kidney transplantation were recently decreased in our hospital by approximately 50%. This led to a considerable decrease of the morbidity rate without a decrease of graft survival (1,2). This change in our immunosuppressive regimen was one reason to undertake an analysis of factors contributing to an increased infection rate after cadaveric kidney transplantation.

PATIENTS

In the Leiden University Hospital, 40-50 cadaveric kidney grafts per year are performed under the auspices of Eurotransplant. The average HLA A+B mismatch is ± 1 and the averaged Dr mismatch is ± 1. For immunosuppression, use is made of prednisone and azathioprine. Patients are nursed in an open ward. Antibiotic prophylaxis is given for all surgical procedures.

One-year patient survival and one-year graft survival amoun to approximately 95% and 75%, respectively.

RESULTS

Between 1977 and 1981, 147 patients received a cadaveric kidney graft. There were 149 infections within the first 3 month after transplantation in 98 patients. No infection developed in 49 patients (33%).

Table I.

TYPES OF INFECTION OBSERVED IN THE FIRST 3 MONTHS AFTER TRANSPLANTATION

	n	%
Urinary tract	53	35
Wound	26	18*
Bacteremia	24	16
Respiratory tract	16	11
Virus	30	20
	149	

* 4% primary infections

Most of the infections occurred in the urinary tract (Table I). A virus infection developed in 20% of the patients, and most of these infections were due to cytomegalo virus.

Several factors were found to give a significant increase in the number of infections. Urinary leakage almost invariably led to an infection. Surgical re-intervention was accompanied by an increased risk of infection. High-dose corticosteroids as well as seronegativity for CMV were associated with an increased infection rate. The influence of a less aggressive rejection therapy and low-dose corticosteroids on the frequency of infections is shown in Table II.

From 1979 onward, rejection treatments were started later, and were also applied less frequently (2.7 versus 1.2). This change of policy led to a decrease of the dose of corticosteroids: from 4.9 g to 3.8 g prednisone and 2.7 g to 0.7 g methylprednisolone. The number of infections decreased from 63 to 33, and the percentage of patients without an infection rose from 18 to 53%. Graft survival was not influenced by the lowering of the dosage of corticosteroids.

Table II.

INFLUENCE OF LESS AGGRESSIVE REJECTION THERAPY AND LOW-DOSE CORTICOSTEROIDS ON THE FREQUENCY OF INFECTIONS IN PATIENTS WITH A FUNCTIONING CADAVERIC KIDNEY GRAFT AFTER 3 MONTHS

	1977/1978 n = 49	1978/1980 n = 57
Start of first rejection treatment, in days	7.2	13.6
Rejection treatments/patient	2.7	1.2
Dose (g) prednisone/patient	4.9 ± 0.9	3.8 ± 1.1
Dose (g) methylprednisolone/ patient	2.7 ± 2.9	0.7 ± 1.3
Number of infections	63	33
Per cent patients without an infection	18	53
Per cent one-year graft survival	75	80

Of the patients with a clinical syndrome associated with CMV infection, 70% received 3 or fewer than 3 blood transfusions before transplantation and were seronegative for CMV. A significant influence was exerted by the number of blood transfusions before transplantation and the percentage of patients who were seropositive for CMV. Of the patients who received up to 3 transfusions, 28% were seropositive compared with 70% of the patients who received more than 10 transfusions.

DISCUSSION

The decrease in the amount of administered corticosteroids by approximately 50% within the first 3 months after transplantation led to a considerable decrease in the number of infection within 3 months. This decrease of the corticosteroid dosage was probably made possible by the optimal grade of histocompatibility between donors and recipient, which is consistent with our findings that less corticosteroid was required by patients who received a well-matched kidney graft (3). The amount of corticosteroids administered in our series of patients was cosiderably lower than that applied in most European centres with the same histocompatibility grade. These differences in immunosuppressive regimens reflect the neglect of research on corticosteroid therapy. Systematic studies on corticosteroids therapy after kidney transplantation deserve high priority (4).

Primary CMV infection was accompanied by considerable morbidity and mortality rates in this series; for instance, all five patients who died of an infection had a primary CMV infection. In our opinion, one of the major fields of effort should be the prevention of primary CMV infection after kidney transplantation. One of the possibilities to prevent primary CMV infection after transplantation might be the induction of a CMV infection while the patient is on dialysis, since in dialysis patients a CMV infection generally runs a benign subclinical course. We therefore advocate planned blood transfusions with fresh blood of CMV-positive donors. In this way, potential recipients of a kidney transplant receive blood transfusions before transplantation for the induction of the so-called transfusion effect (5).

REFERENCES

1. Hooff van, J.P., Es van, A., Koolen, M.I., Kalff, M.W., Broek van den, P.J., Graeff de, J. 1980. Less aggressive rejection therapy and low-dose corticosteroids leading to satisfactory cadaveriĉ kidney graft survival and low morbidity rate. Proc. Eur. Dial. Transplant Assoc. 17: 435.
2. Henstra, G, Hooff van, J.P. 1980. Less aggressive rejection therapy and low-dose corticosteroids leading to a change in nursing aspects of cadaveric kidney transplantation. Proc. Eur. Dial. Transplant Assoc. 8: 96.
3. Hooff van, J.P., Hooff van-Eykenboom, I.J.E.A., Kalff, M.W., Graeff de, J., Rood van, J.J. 1979. Kidney graft survival: Clincial course and HLA, A,B, and D matching in 208 patients transplanted in one centre. Transplant. Proc. XI: 1291.
4. Hooff van, J.P. 1980. Priorities in transplantation research Lancet i: 43.
5. Hooff van, J.P., Kalff, M.W., Poelgeest van, A.E., Persyn, G.G., Rood van, J.J. 1976. Bloodtransfusions and kidney transplantation. Transplantation 22: 306.

DISCUSSION EDITED BY J.P. VAN HOOFF

van Furth: Dr. Rubin, would you like to comment on Dr. van Hooff's questions, for instance about low-dose immunosuppression, the poor outcome of primary CMV infection, and vaccination against CMV infection with planned blood transfusions?

Rubin: It is probably the benificial effect of HLA-matching that allows certain centres in Europe to use such low dosages for immunosuppression. It is difficult to demonstrate this beneficial effect of matching in the USA. This lack of influence of matching might be due to the more heterogeneous ethnic population of the USA, as has been suggested by the Leiden group. Therefore, it might be impossible to lower the dosages of corticosteroids considerably in the USA. I completely agree with Dr. van Hooff about the bad prognosis of a primary CMV infection after kidney transplantation. We have recently analysed the data of 1,600 renal transplant patients from 41 centres in the USA, and concluded that those patients who were at risk for developing primary CMV had an increased rate of death, of graft loss, and of grafts with a poor function.

I think the suggestion made by Dr. van Hooff about vaccination against CMV via planned blood transfusions is a wonderful idea. There is no question that it would be an excellent way to make these patients CMV seropositive. However, what bothers me is that with transfusions one sensitizes the patient against histocompatibility antigens. This sensitization will lead to a decrease in the number of suitable kidneys for these patients. An alternative approach might be the use of CMV vaccine, but unfortunately a suitable vaccine will not be available on a large scale within the next few years. Recently, we have been working with human interferon prophylaxis and have found that it was leading to a decrease of the incidence of reactivation of CMV.

van Hooff: We transfuse our patients, because if patients are not given a transfusion before transplantation the graft has a very bad outcome. The optimal number of transfusions is probably about three, and with this number of transfusions the risk of sensitization is low. I advocate the selection of donors who are positive for CMV and the use of their blood for induction of not only the transfusion effect but also to make the patients seropositive for CMV.

van Furth: Dr. van Hooff, if you introduce a CMV infection into a dialysis population, this might lead to an increased chance of reactivation after transplantation.

van Hooff: I completely agree with you, but a reactivation after transplantation generally has a good prognosis and reactivation was relatively rare in our patients. I want to stress the importance of preventing the development of a primary CMV infection after transplantation, because of the serious complications associated with such infection.

Rubin: Patients who are at risk for a primary CMV infection have a roughly 70% chance of getting into trouble, whereas of the patients who are at risk for reactivation, only 20% will get into trouble. So by giving transfusion with CMV you might convert your 70% risk into about 20% risk.

van Furth: I wonder whether the solution might be the transfusion of frozen leucocytes.

van Hooff: That would mean the loss of the beneficial effect of blood transfusions on kidney-graft survival.

Weimar: In recent years we have been very careful with the dosages used for immunosuppression. When there is a life-threatening infection, azathioprine and prednisone are stopped. Since this change, our death rate has decreased from 14% to nil. Graft survival after one year was unaltered.

Rubin: Since we adopted a similar approach a couple of years ago, infection is no longer the major cause of death.

van Hooff: We have been seeing relatively very few opportunistic infections in our patients, compared with Dr. Rubin's series. Is that the result of the low-dose immunosuppression or are there other factors involved as well?

Rubin: I do not think that this difference is due solely to immunosuppression. In my opinion, epidemiological factors are of importance as well; for example, we had an epidemic of pseudomonas pneumonia. It turned out that the pseudomonas came via the ventilation system directly to the patient. This underlines the importance of nosocomial hazards.

van der Meer: Pneumococcal pneumonia has been leading to a high morbidity rate in our transplant patients. We have not yet decided whether to vaccinate these patients. Dr. Rubin, do you have any data about the efficacy of vaccination?

Rubin: We are vaccinating the dialysis patients. It is clear that induction of immunity is not nearly as good as in a normal individual: for instance, we have observed pneumococcal infection in immunosuppressed patients who have received the pneumococcal vaccine.

van der Meer: Dr. Young suggested that Pneumocystis carinii pneumonia is due to reactivation in patients already harbouring pneumocystis. I got the impression that you did not exclude the possibility of an exogenous source.

Rubin: I think reactivation is probably the major factor, although there is circumstantial evidence which suggests there might be an exogenous source as well; for example, there has been clustering of patients with pneumocystis infections in several hospitals.

In corticosteroid-treated animals there is a possibility of transmission of the pneumocystis via the air. In two different hospitals in Boston which were using similar immunosuppressive regimens for a similar patient population, we found that there was a significant difference in the incidence of pneumocystis infections. Because of this circumstantial evidence, I still remain concerned about the possibility of nosocomial clustering through some kind of person-to-person spread. It is our policy that we isolate such patients from other immunosuppressed individuals, although we realize that this policy is not based on a well-controlled study.

COST-BENEFIT ASPECTS OF SURVEILLANCE OF HOSPITAL INFECTIONS

R.W. HALEY

Resources have never been abundant for the support of disease prevention programs, and today's worldwide economic problems render such funding even more scarce. Consequently, decision makers at the national, state and individual-hospital levels are forced to choose among numerous alternative programs that compete for the precious available resources. One of the valuable tools used in this decision-making process is the comparison of the costs of a preventive program with its expected benefits, often referred to as cost-benefit analysis.

In the prevention of nosocomial infections in the United States, one of the central elements in our approach is the adoption of organized infection surveillance and control programs (ISCPs) in individual hospitals. These programs basically involve the employment of a full- or part-time infection control nurse who performs surveillance of infections and works with an infection control committee, and perhaps with a physician epidemiologist, to formulate and carry out various infection control and prevention measures. Almost all U.S. hospitals now have such surveillance programs in operation (1). In contrast to other disease prevention programs which may at least partially support themselves financially (e.g., immunization programs, cancer screening clinics), ISCPs represent only a cost to hospitals but generate no direct revenue from patients or their insurance carriers. Decision makers in hospitals (e.g., hospital administrators) are often reluctant to dedicate resources to infection surveillance and control in the face of seriously constrained operating budgets. This circumstance probably explains the widespread attention given to the cost-benefit analysis of infection control in the literature of this field.

Although much has been written on this subject in the last decade, there are still many misconceptions about the methods of cost-benefit analysis and its proper applications. In this paper, I will introduce a set of cost-benefit figures derived several years ago, survey the literature briefly, evaluate some alternative methods of estimating the costs of nosocomial infections, and discuss some of the important factors that determine the magnitude of these costs, including the need to identify high-cost nosocomial infections. The purpose of this report is to raise a number of issues that should be understood in future evaluations of the costs and benefits of infection control.

A PRELIMINARY COST-BENEFIT ANALYSIS

In the mid 1970s as part of a larger program to avaluate the efficacy of ISCPs, I developed a preliminary cost-benefit analysis to serve as the basis for project planning (2). To summarize the argument, of the approximately 34 million patients admitted to general hospitals in the United States each year (3), about 5 % develop a nosocomial infection (4, 5), accounting for approximately 1.7 million nosocomial infections per year. Assuming that each infection adds approximately $ 600 to the patient's hospitalization costs (6), the excess hospital costs due to nosocomial infections amounted to approximately one billion dollars in 1971 (Table 1).

Table 1.
ESTIMATED ANNUAL COSTS OF NOSOCOMIAL INFECTIONS

34,000,000	Patient admissions, community hospitals
X .05	Proportion of patients with nosocomial infection
1,700,000	Estimated number of patients with nosocomial infections
X $ 600	Average extra routine and ancillary charges per infection
$ 1,020,000,000	Excess hospital charges due to nosocomial infections

Adjusting this figure for the approximately 12 % rate of inflation of hospital costs per year since 1976, we would estimate the excess hospital costs due to nosocomial infections at about 2 billion dollars in 1982.

Table 2.
ESTIMATED ANNUAL COSTS OF ISCPs

A. Itemized Cost of an ISCP for each 250 Hospital Beds		
	$ 12,000	One infection control nurse
	5,000	Hospital epidemiologist (physician, part-time)
	2,000	Clerical assistance (1/4 time at $ 8,000 annual salary)
+	1,000	Miscellaneous expenses
	$ 20,000	Cost of an ISCP for 250 hospital beds
B. Cost of ISCPs Nationwide		
	898,000	Community hospital beds in U.S.
-	250	Beds per ISCP
	3,592	ISCPs needed for all community hospitals
X	$ 20,000	Cost per ISCP (From A. above)
	$ 71,840,000	Cost for all community hospitals

To estimate the costs of the prevention program, I estimated the cost of employing a full-time infection control nurse, a part-time hospital epidemiologist, clerical assistance and other miscellaneous expenses to be about $ 20,000 for every 250 beds (7) (Table 2). Since there are 898,000 community hospital beds in the United States, the cost of establishing and maintaining ISCPs in all U.S. hospitals would have amounted to approximately 71 million dollars in 1976 (Table 2). Dividing the costs of the prevention programs (Table 2) by the total costs of the infections (Table 1) gives a cost-benefit ratio of 6.3 %, indicating that if the prevention programs decreased the extra hospital costs of the infections by only 6.3 % there would be sufficient savings to finance completely all infection control programs in the country. Any additional reduction beyond the 6.3 % would produce a net economic benefit from the programs.

From preliminary studies in several individual hospitals (8), it seems likely that an ongoing ISCP might maintain the nosocomial infection rate 20 % to 50 % lower than it would be without the program. From the cost-benefit relationship, we can estimate the net benefits at three levels of infection control program effectiveness (Table 3). If the programs reduce the cost of infections by 6.3 %, roughly 100,000 patients would be spared the morbidity, mortality, and costs of nosocomial infections, and from a financial standpoint the program would be in approximate cost-benefit balance.

Table 4.
ANNUAL BENEFITS OF ISCPs AT THREE LEVELS OF CONTROL EFFECTIVENESS

	Assumed Reduction of Nosocomial Infections		
	6.3 %	20 %	50 %
Patients in whom infections were prevented	100,184	316,710	791,775
Gross benefit	$ 71,840,000	$ 227,106,000	$ 567,766,000
Cost of ISCPs	$ 71,840,000	$ 71,840,000	$ 71,840,000
NET BENEFIT	$ 0	$ 155,266,000	$ 495,926,000

If the programs prevent 20 % of the costs, 300,000 patients would be spared from infections, representing a saving of over $ 150 million dollars per year. Similarly a 50 % rate of effectiveness would spare more than 3/4 of a million patients from infections and save more than 1/2 billion dollars per year.

This abbreviated analysis raises many questions. By far the most important concerns the degree of reduction of nosocomial infections by ISCPs. If indeed the prevention amounts to 20 % or more of the costs of infections, ISCPs will clearly provide a net benefit regardless of the means of resolving other problems in the cost-benefit technique. To address this prevention question, we have been conducting a nationwide study, called the SENIC Project (Study on the Efficacy of Nosocomial Infection Control), in a random sample of U.S. hospitals to estimate the percentage of nosocomial infections prevented by ISCPs. A preliminary report provided encouraging evidence on this question, but we have yet to complete the analyses to provide definitive evidence of this preventive effect (9).

A second methodological problem illustrated by this example involves confusion over what costs should be included in the total costs of maintaining an ISCP. I chose to include only those costs required to perform surveillance of infections and to manage the control and prevention efforts. It can be argued that the program costs should include the costs of all diagnostic, therapeutic and other aspects of patient care practiced to prevent infection (e.g., sterile closed system urinary drainage systems, prophylactic antibiotics, and private rooms for isolation). The counter argument attests that, since these patient-care practices are minimal standards of care and should be practiced in all hospitals, they should not be included in the costs of ISCPs.

Certainly the most difficult aspect of this type of analysis is the estimation of the costs of nosocomial infections. The first complication arises from the fact that hospital charges, which represent the most readily measurable source of data, may not necessarily reflect actual hospital costs for treating the infections. This disparity arises from the complex billing systems of hospitals in which the costs of some services for which hospitals cannot charge directly may be recovered by charging excessively for other services (10). As yet, no studies have estimated the true hospital costs of nosocomial infections, and we must presently be content with estimates based on hospital charges. One way of avoiding this issue is to use extra hospital days attributable to nosocomial infection in place of hospital costs. This has proved unsatisfactory, however, in two respects : first, there are serious methodological difficulties in estimating extra days of hospitalization, and second, limiting the analysis to extra days ignores the costly impact of hospital services and other ancillary costs that may vary independent of extra days.

ESTIMATING THE COST OF NOSOCOMIAL INFECTIONS

In the past, two different approaches have been taken for the estimation of extra days and extra costs attributable to nosocomial infections. In the earliest studies, these were estimated directly by physicians who observed infected patients daily to determine which days were actually due to nosocomial infection ; examples of physicians' direct assessments of prolongation of stay due to surgical wound infections are shown in Table 5.

Table 5.
SUMMARY OF RESULTS OF STUDIES THAT ATTEMPTED TO ESTIMATE THE EXTRA DAYS OR DOLLAR COSTS OF NOSOCOMIAL INFECTIONS BY PHYSICIAN'S ESTIMATE

Study (reference)	Last year of study period	Average extra days (extra cost)		
		ALL	SWI	BACT*
Eliason and McLaughlin (11)	1933	--	6.75-11.2	--
Goodall (12)	1950	21	--	--
Clarke (13)	1953	--	1.36	--
Public Health Laboratory Service (14)	1959	--	7.5	--
Haley et al. (15)	1975	4.5 ($ 590)	8.2 ($ 884)	9.4 ($ 903)

* ALL = all nosocomial infections ;
SWI = surgical wound infections ;
BACT = nosocomial bacteremia

In later years, medical scientists, noting that the earlier estimates were "uncontrolled studies", attempted to estimate the extra days (and charges) by comparing the average length of stay (and total hospital charges) of nosocomially infected patients with that of non-infected patients, who served as "controls". Subtracting the former from the latter yielded an estimate of the prolongation of stay and extra charges (Table 6).

Recognizing that patients destined to develop nosocomial infections were often more seriously ill, and thus already destined to stay longer in the hospital, than non-infected patients, other investigators attempted to match a non-infected "control" patient with each infected patient on characteristics that predispose to nosocomial infection. It was argued that a matched case-control analysis would reduce the bias from differences in the degree of underlying illness and yield more accurate estimates of extra days and charges. Although it is difficult to compare the various studies on account of differences in the types of patients and infections studied, the results suggest that the case-control comparison studies yielded estimates of extra days 2-3 times higher than the physicians' direct assessment method and that this difference was only slightly reduced when matching was employed (Tables 5 and 6).

Table 6.

SUMMARY OF RESULTS OF STUDIES THAT ATTEMPTED TO ESTIMATE THE EXTRA DAYS OR DOLLAR COSTS OF NOSOCOMIAL INFECTIONS BY COMPARING INFECTED AND UNINFECTED PATIENTS

Study (reference)	Last year of study period	Were Controls Matched ?	Extra days (extra cost)		
			ALL	SWI	BACT*
Clarke (13)	1953	No	--	5	--
Lowenthal (16)	1960	Yes	--	7.3	--
Fekety (17)	1965	Yes	--	18	--
Thoburn et al. (18)	1966	No	--	14.1-26.3	--
Speery and Craddock (19)	1966	Yes	--	15.2 (669)	--
Amer. Coll. Surgeons (20)	1970	No	--	23.87 (2,387)	--
Westwood et al. (21)	1972	No	22 (1,650)		--
Simchen and Sacks (22)	1973	Yes	--		--
Freeman et al. (23)	1973	Yes	3		--
Spengler and Greenough (24)	1974	Yes	--		14 (3,600)
Rose et al. (25)	1974	Yes	--		32 (4,370)
Green and Wenzel (26)	1975	Yes	--	7.8 (987)	--
Haley et.al. (15)	1975	Yes	13.4 (1,018)	10.2 (775)	14.0 (1,064)

* ALL = all nosocomial infections ;
SWI = surgical wound infections ;
BACT = nosocomial bacteremia

Suspecting that the controlled studies might have been substantially overestimating the extra days, in 1975 we performed a pilot study at Grady Memorial Hospital in Atlanta, Georgia, to compare the three methods by performing them on the same group of patients. The methods and results of this study have been published (15) and will only be summarized here. Basically, a physician epidemiologist visited each patient with a nosocomial infection daily to determine which, if any, days of hospitalization were attributable primarily to the infection and to record all ancillary services and costs required each day for treating the infection. Later, he reviewed each infected patient's itemized hospital bill to obtain the actual charges for each extra day and for all services attributable to infection. From these data we calculated the average extra days and charges representing the physician's direct assessment.

Following the prospective data collection phase, we employed two case-control methods to estimate these same parameters. First, we analyzed the computerized data file to match a non-infected patient to each infected patient on the basis of exact primary diagnosis, first surgical procedure, second surgical procedure, age, sex and service. We then calculated the difference in length of stay between the two members of each pair and averaged the differences over all matched pairs to obtain an estimate of the extra days attributable to infection by the matched comparison method. Second, we repeated the case-control study without matching by simply subtracting the average length of stay of all infected patients from that of all non-infected patients to obtain an estimate of extra days by the case-control method without matching. In this pilot study, we enrolled 4,067 consecutive admissions among whom we discovered 211 patients with nosocomial infection ; of these, we studied 183 whose itemized hospital bills could be located. For 120 of these patients we were able to identify a non-infected patient matched exactly on the matching criteria and 58 more who were matched "closely", leaving five infected patients for whom a matched control could not be found.

Table 7.

COMPARISON OF RESULTS FROM THREE METHODS OF ESTIMATING AVERAGE EXTRA DAYS AND CHARGES ATTRIBUTABLE TO NOSOCOMIAL INFECTION

Parameter estimated	Physician's Assessment	Comparison Method	
		Matched	Not Matched
Days	4.8	13.4	16.7
Routine charges ($)	357	1,018	1,269
Ancillary charges ($)	219	--	--
Total charges ($)	576	--	--

Analysis of these data revealed that estimates of extra days were three and a half times higher by the non-matched case-control method than by the physician's assessment and that this disparity was reduced only slightly by matching (Table 7). The extra routine charges associated with the extra days bore a similar relationship. This difference between estimates by the different methods held true when analyzed by the service on which the patients were hospitalized and for infections occurring at most sites (15).

In trying to determine whether this difference between the physician's assessment and the matched comparison methods was due to residual bias in the matching procedure, we performed further analyses to see whether the infected patients may have been more seriously ill to begin with than their matched controls. Indeed, we found that infected patients underwent, on the average more surgical operations than their matched controls (mean 1.2 vs. 1.0 operations per patient, $p = 0.10$) and had more discharge diagnoses recorded (mean 2.5 vs. 2.1 per patient, $p = 0.02$). Although the differences were not statistically significant, the infected patients were also more likely to have had their hospitalization complicated by a pulmonary embolus, acute renal failure, and death in the hospital. Thus, we concluded that the case-control method, even when patients were matched for characteristics that predispose to infection, was seriously biased by a disparity in the degree of underlying illness.

At this point, it appears that the physician's direct assessment may be the most accurate of the three present alternatives for estimating the extra days and costs, although there is some reason to suspect that it may somewhat underestimate these parameters and it is much more difficult and time-consuming to perform. We are currently investigating a new method of estimation in which we match infected patients with groups of controls on the basis of a complex model that predicts underlying predisposition to lengthy hospital stay. It appears that controlling for predictors of length of stay, rather than for predictors of infection risk alone, may give the most accurate estimates.

DETERMINANTS OF THE COST OF NOSOCOMIAL INFECTIONS

To study the determinants of the cost of nosocomial infections, we enrolled two more hospitals of different types into the pilot studies and estimated the extra days and costs due to nosocomial infections in these hospitals by the physician's assessment method exactly as performed in the first hospital. The methods used and the characteristics of the hospitals have been published elsewhere (6). By comparing the results, we found remarkably few differences among the three hospitals. Nosocomial infections on the average accounted for extra days per infection of 4.5, 3.7 and 3.1 in the three hospitals, respectively, and for extra charges per infection of $ 590, $ 598 and $ 641, respectively. Although these average figures varied little among the hospitals, there was a wide range of total extra charges among patients, the highest being $ 12,261 and 112 extra days.

A second remarkable finding was that the extra charges were divided about equally between the extra routine charges ("per diem charges") billed automatically for the extra days and the ancillary charges billed for specific diagnostic and therapeutic services required to treat the infection. This finding indicates that past studies confined only to estimates of extra days may underestimate the total costs of nosocomial infections by as much as 50 %. However, we found marked differences in the extra days and extra charges attributable to nosocomial infection related to the site of infection, the service to which the patient was admitted, the sequence of infection when a patient contracted more than one, and the development of secondary bacteremia. Specifically, the extra days and costs attributable to nosocomial respiratory tract infections, surgical wound infections and primary bacteremia were substantially higher than for urinary tract infections and other types of infection (e.g., nursery-acquired pyoderma). They were also substantially higher for patients admitted to the medicine and surgery services than for those admitted to gynecology, obstetrics, pediatrics, and the newborn service, although the differences by service did not remain statistically significant when controlling for the differences by site of infection. Nosocomial infections complicated by secondary bacteremia were about 3 1/2 times more costly than those without secondary bacteremia, and this relationship held for all types of infection except for lower respiratory infections.

Perhaps the most remarkable finding was that a relatively small proportion of the infected patients accounted for a disproportionately large share of the total extra costs attributable to nosocomial infections in the three hospitals. Specifically, we found that the 10 % of patients with the highest total extra charges accounted for 38 %, 46 % and 65 % of all nosocomial infection costs in the three hospitals, respectively, and 25 % of the patients accounted for 64 %, 72 % and 86 %, respectively. This finding is quite important since it indicates that preventive efforts aimed at a relatively small group of patients might prevent the great majority of extra days and costs of nosocomial infections.

We have recently extended these analyses to identify, if possible, combinations of characteristics, available early in hospitalization, that would identify groups of patients at high risk for the most costly nosocomial infections. An initial report (27) suggests that most of these high-cost infections occur on the medicine and surgery services. Of particular importance are cases of nosocomial pneumonia on the medicine service and surgical wound infections, especially in patients with traumatic injuries, on the surgery service. An important next question is whether these high-cost infections are preventable. If they are not, we will have identified questions of high priority for basic or applied research. If they are, we might be able to confine much of our infection surveillance and control effort to such groups of patients susceptible to the high-cost nosocomial infections and thereby improve the cost-benefit ratio of our prevention efforts.

REFERENCES

1. Haley, R.W., Shachtman, R.H. 1981. The emergence of infection surveillance and control programs in U.S. hospitals : An assessment, 1976. Am. J. Epidemiol. 111 : 574.
2. Haley, R.W. Preliminary Cost-Benefit Analysis of Hospital Infection Control Programs (The SENIC Project). 1977. Proceedings of an International Workshop at Baiersbronn, West Germany. Ed. Franz Daschner. Gustav Fischer Verlag, Stuttgart, 93.
3. American Hospital Association. 1976. Guide to the health care field. Chicago : American Hospital Association.
4. Bennett, J.V., Scheckler, Maki, D.G., Brachman, P.S. 1971. Current national patterns : United States. In : Proceedings of the International Conference on Nosocomial Infections, Atlanta, Georgia, Center for Disease Control, August 3-6, 1970. Chicago, IL : American Hospital Association, 42.
5. Haley, R.W., Hooton, T.M., Culver, D.H., et al. 1981. Nosocomial infections in U.S. hospitals, 1975-1976 : estimated frequency by selected characteristics of patients. Am. J. Med. 70 : 947.
6. Haley, R.W., Schaberg, D.R., Von Allmen, S.A., McGowan, J.E. Jr. 1981. Estimating the extra charges and prolongation of hospitalization due to nosocomial infections : a comparison of methods. J. Infect. Dis. 141 : 248.
7. Center for Disease Control. 1970. Outline for the surveillance and control of nosocomial infections. CDC, Atlanta, Georgia.
8. Shoji, K.T., Axnick, K., Rytel, M.W. 1974. Infections and antibiotic use in a large municipal hospital 1970-1972 : a prospective analysis of the effectiveness of a continuous surveillance program. Health Lab. Sci. 11 : 283.
9. Haley, R.W., Culver, D.H., Emori, T.G., et al. 1981. Progress report on the evaluation of the efficacy of infection surveillance and control programs. Am. J. Med. 70 : 971.

10. Finkler, S.A. 1982. The distinction between costs and charges. Ann. Intern. Med. 96 : 102.
11. Eliason, E.L., McLaughlin, C. 1934. Post-operative wound complications. Annals of Surgery 100 : 1159.
12. Goodall, J.W.D. 1952. Cross-infection in hospital wards : its incidence and prevention. Lancet 1 : 807.
13. Clark, S.K.R. 1957. Sepsis in surgical wounds, with particular reference to Staphylococcus aureus. Br. J. Surg. 44 : 592.
14. Public Health Laboratory Service. 1960. Incidence of surgical wound infection in England and Wales. Lancet 2 : 659.
15. Haley, R.W., Schaberg, D.R., Crossley, K.B., Von Allmen, S.A., McGowan, J.E. Jr. 1981. Extra Charges and prolongation of hospitalization due to nosocomial infections : a prospective interhospital comparison. Am. J. Med. 70 : 51.
16. Lowenthal, J. 1962. Sources and sequelae of surgical sepsis. Br. Med. J. 1 : 1437.
17. Fekety, F.R. 1965. The epidemiology of infections in surgical patients. In B.S. Berlin and M. Hilbert (ed.). Control of infections in hospitals. Proceedings of an institute, University of Michigan, March 1-3, 1965. University of Michigan School of Public Health, Continuing Education Service, Ann Arbor, 24.
18. Thoburn, R., Fekety, F.R., Cluff, L.E., Melvin, V.B. 1968. Infections acquired by hospitalized patients. Archives of Internal Medicine 121 : 1.
19. Sperry, H.E., Craddock, J. 1968. It pays to spend money for infection control. Mod. Hosp. 111 : 124.
20. Committee on Control of Surgical Infections of the Committee on Pre- and Post-operative Care, American College of Surgeons. 1976. Manual on control of infection in surgical patients. J.B. Lippincott Co., Philadelphia, 11.
21. Westwood, J.C.N., Legrace, S., Mitchell, M.A. 1974. Hospital-acquired infection : present and future impact and need for positive action. Can. Med. Assoc. J. 110 : 769.
22. Simchen, E., Sacks, T. 1975. Infection in war wounds-experience during the 1973 October war in Israel. Ann. Surg. 182 : 754.
23. Freeman, J., Rosner, B.A., McGowan J.E. Jr. 1979. Adverse effects of nosocomial infection. J. Infect. Dis. 140 : 732.
24. Spengler, R.F., Greenough, W.B. 1978. Hospital costs and mortality attributed to nosocomial bacteremias. JAMA 240 : 2455.
25. Rose, R., Hunting, K.J., Townsend, T.R., Wenzel, R.P. 1977. Morbidity/mortality and economics of hospital-acquired blood stream infections : a controlled study. South. Med. J. 70 : 1267.
26. Green, J.W., Wenzel, R.P. 1977. Postoperative wound infection : a controlled study of the increased duration of hospital stay and direct cost of hospitalization. Annals of Surgery 185 : 264.

27. Pinner, R.W., Haley, R.W., Blumenstein, D.A., Schaberg, D.R., Von Allmen, S.D., McGowan, J.E. Jr. 1982. High cost nosocomial infections. Infect. Contr. 3 : 143.

COMMENTS ON ISSUES IN STUDYING THE COST-BENEFIT OF HOSPITAL INFECTION SURVEILLANCE AND CONTROL PROGRAMS

J.I. HUDSON

The ultimate value of cost-benefit analysis lies in the potential for its use in the decision making process when one is confronted with competing strategies in the face of finite resources. In the case of nosocomial infection surveillance, the quest for 'best' strategy can be enhanced by cost-benefit analysis provided that the right questions are asked, valid and reliable data are generated to establish prohabilities, and sensible interpretations of the data are made. Here, three groups of questions emerge : (a) given finite resources, where do we concentrate efforts ? (cost-benefit enquiry) ; (b) having once established the target, which method should be employed ? (cost-effectiveness, systems analysis exercise) ; (c) once a program has been initiated, how do we monitor its benefit relative to the input costs ? (combined cost-benefit, cost-effectiveness issue).

Recently a number of well-designed studies have provided us with partial answers to the three orders of questions. First, through carefully managed incidence studies by Haley and his co-workers (1), we know that - in the U.S. hospital population - about one in 10 general medical and surgical patients will have at least one nosocomial infection at one or more of the four major sites (urinary tract, surgical wound, lower respiratory tract, bloodstream, and that approximately seven out of ten of these infections will be found in surgical patients. Roughly similar findings were recently reported from the National Survey of Infections in Hospitals in the U.K. (2). Extensive cost analysis studies conducted by Haley and others (3) have identified the most costly infections in terms of resource expenditures and prolongation of the hospital stay.

These are : cases of secondary bacteremia complicating already acquired nosocomial infections, lower respiratory tract infections, and surgical wound infections. These cost studies demonstrate clearly that a relatively small number of patients, between 10 % and 20 % of those who acquire a hospital infection, account for about 50 % of the total extra charges attributable to nosocomial infections.

Thus, while we may find it prudent - e.g. : cost-effective - to maintain general surveillance/control for all patients following guidelines published here (4) and elsewhere (5), we now have a good "lead" on a high-risk group of patients where it may be especially worthwhile to concentrate our efforts. We need to search for more information on the intrinsic characteristics of this small high-cost group, particularly as it relates to effective surveillance and control methods.

The second order question requires an enquiry into the most efficient surveillance/control methods to apply to this group. Data under analysis by Haley and co-workers in the Study on the Efficacy of Nosocomial Infection Control (SENIC Project) (6) may well provide some answers. For example, detailed analysis in which some of the important confounding variables are controlled appears to show a powerful positive correlation between focused surveillance and control programs and a reduced incidence of nosocomial infections (7). If these preliminary findings are confirmed by further analysis of the data, it will mean that, when applied vigorously, focused surveillance and control works. Further refinements of the method should include more accurate estimation of the true hospital costs of caring for nosocomial infections (rather than using patient charges as a proxy) and perhaps further standardization of the definitions of attributable extra days and services. What will be needed then is further developmental research to help determine just which specific methods are most effective under varying conditions.

Some headway is also being made towards a more objective method of program evaluation, the third order question, again thanks to some meticulous investigations by Haley and co-workers.

The measurement of direct costs of the program is relatively straightforward. What has always been a problem is the estimate of the direct medical costs, in terms of resource expenditures, increased hospital days, etc., which are theoretically avoided through successful surveillance and control. A uniform method for the estimation of such direct cost savings has been developed and tested (8), and its application to on-going cost-benefit monitoring seems promising. Those of us interested in quality assurance in general can see the usefulness of this methodology for program impact evaluation.

There are two other correlations with general quality assurance activities that now seem obvious. First, when considering the entire spectrum of patients admitted to acute care hospitals, it appears that a relatively small number, between 10 % - 15 %, generate a disproportionately large share, over 50 %, of the total yearly hospital charges (9-11). It is tempting to speculate that this group might represent a prime, high pay-off target for quality assurance and risk management activities. This speculation is made all the more attractive in light of studies which identify a higher incidence of iatrogenic illnesses (12) and surgical mishaps (13) in this very group of high-risk patients. Applying some crude mathematics combining these data with those from the studies by Haley and co-workers in 1976, the incidence study in England and Wales in 1980, and Haley's cost analysis study, one comes up with the estimate that nosocomial infections constitute the major problem in approximately 0.3 % of all high-cost patients. Three tenths of one percent seems a very small figure. For proper perspective, however, we need to know what proportion of these high costs are potentially and easily prevented. This information is not available from the high-cost patient studies reported to date. Such an investigative analysis across discriminate diagnostic-severity groupings stands out as a clear high priority on the immediate health services research, quality assurance agenda.

Finally, there is the matter of what Richard Dixon (14), a former colleague of Dr Haley's, describes as the "missing link" in hospital infection control : translating the understanding about nosocomial infections and the knowledge about how to prevent them into standardized, routine practice. This conference has yielded a number of excellent and timely papers on the epidemiology of hospital infections. This last paper - on the cost-benefit of surveillance - begins to forge that missing link ; it transcends the areas of epidemiology and quality evaluation ; it begins to answer the question, what methods are effective, and how can we assure their efficient application ? The next question asks : given effective methods and an efficient means, how well are we applying these in our local situation ? What is the potential for improvement ? This, of course, is the heart of quality assurance. The deliberate integration of effective and efficient surveillance/ control mechanisms with comprehensive, hospitalwide quality assurance programs is a goal well within our reach and certainly deserving of our immediate attention.

REFERENCES

1. Haley, R.W., Hooton, T.M., Culver, D.H., et al. 1981. Nosocomial Infections in U.S. Hospitals, 1975-1976. Estimated Frequency by Selected Characteristics of Patients. Am. J. Med. 70 : 947.
2. Meers, P.D., Ayliffe, G.A.L., Emmerson, A.M., et al. 1981. Report on the National Survey of Infection in Hospitals, 1980. J. hosp. Infection. 2 : Supplement. 51.
3. Haley, R.W., Schaberg, D.R., Crossley, K.B., Von Allmen, S.A., McGowan, J.E. Jr. 1981. Extra Charges and Prolongation of Stay Attributable to Nosocomial Infections : A Prospective Interhospital Comparison. Am. J. Med. 70 : 51.
4. Preventing Hospital Infections. Guidelines proposed by the Health Council of the Netherlands. Ministry of Health and Environmental Protection. 1980.
5. Guidelines for the Prevention and Control of Nosocomial Infections. Hospital Infections Branch. CDC. Atlanta, 1981.
6. Haley, R.W., Culver, D.H., Emori, T.G., et al. 1981. Progress Report on the Evaluation of Efficacy of Infection Surveillance and Control Programs. Am. J. Med. 70 : 971.
7. Haley, R.W. Presentation before the Second International Conference on Nosocomial Infections. Atlanta, Georgia, August 5-8, 1980.
8. Haley, R.W., Schaberg, D.R., Von Allmen, S.A., McGowan J.E. Jr. 1981. Estimating the Extra Charges and Prolongation of Hospitalization Due to Nosocomial Infections : A Comparison of Methods. J. Inf. Dis. 141 : 248.

9. Schroeder, S.A., Showstack, J.A., Roberts H.E. 1979. Frequency and Clinical Description of High-Cost Patients in 17 Acute-Care Hospitals. M. Eng. J. Med. 300 : 1306.
10. Schroeder, S.A., Showstack, J.A., Roberts H.E. 1981. Survival of Adult High-Cost Patients. Report of a Follow-up Study from Nine Acute-Care Hospitals. JAMA. 245 : 1446.
11. Zook, C.D., Moore, F.D. 1980. High-Cost Users of Medical Care. N. Eng. J. Med. 302 : 996.
12. Steel, K., Gertman, P.M., Crescenzi, C., Anderson, J. 1981. Iatrogenic Illness on a General Medical Service at a University Hospital. N. Eng. J. Med. 304 : 638.
13. Couch, N.P., Tilney N.L., Rayner, A.A., Moore, F.D. 1981. The High Cost of Low-Frequency Events. The Anatomy and Economics of Surgical Mishaps. N. Eng. J. Med. 304 : 634.
14. Dixon, R.E. 1981. Forging the Missing Link in Infection Control. Am. J. Med. 70 : 976.

DISCUSSION EDITED BY J.I. HUDSON

Mattie: There is a point on which both speakers have dwelt but which has always puzzled me: You do a study like this to prove that the program will pay for itself. In a way, however, the hospital sells services to the patient. Now, if you introduce an infection-control program that diminishes the charges to the patient while the fixed costs for the hospital remain the same, it appears that the hospital will have to absorb the costs that are saved. Who is going to pay for that?

Haley: That is a critical question in the cost-benefit analysis of infection control, i.e., what are the economic incentives for preventing infections in situations where the hospital seemingly increases income by keeping the patient in a long time? There are several answers to this. First, there are certain types of hospital in which nosocomial infections do not increase the hospital's revenue. In the U.S., a sizable proportion of our hospitals are small enterpreneural enterprises run for profit. They tend to do low-risk surgery and turn the patients over very rapidly. Patients usually stay no longer than three to five days, and most of the revenue is generated on the first day. After the initial surgery, the post-operative period generates very low daily revenue, and therefore they try for rapid bed turn-overs. Thus, most of their days are "first-day" days, and they generally have very high occupancy rates, almost 100%. If they have a patient in the hospital for two weeks, they are not getting that big peak of revenue on the first day. It is not to their benefit to have infections. In the majority of U.S. hospitals (non-proprietary), the daily average revenue curve does not fall as rapidly and their occupancy rates are not as high (i.e., more in the range of 75%). Here you might see nosocomial infections keeping patients in the hospital, filling those beds, and in some ways bringing in more revenue. However, these are the types of hospital where the administrators tend to be more motivated by altruism or other professional ethics to reduce infections. Furthermore, I think that if you look carefully into all hospital costs and the revenues, especially the cost of caring for a patient with a nosocomial infection versus the revenue from that patient, you will find that the occurrences of nosocomial infections do not benefit the hospital, because such mishaps often require extra expenditures which are not recovered in the revenue. Finally, the fact that costs do not equal charges really complicates this discussion. The problem is that you often cannot determine the precise influence of extra days on the operating costs. We are starting to look into this issue to determine whether the extra costs associated with nosocomial infections are more (or less) recoverable from direct revenue.

Thus, at this point, the answer to your question is complex. There is a lot to be learned from looking further into this question.

Hudson: I have additonal comments related to that question. The first pertains to a situation in the United States and which may or may not become commonplace here in a few years. That is, the cost of risk-management programs, particularly the insurance, is now so expensive that most hospitals are self-insured. Any sustained reduction of conditions leading to liability will result in direct cost-savings. Finally, those hospitals which are under some sort of prospective budgeting arrangement will, of course, find it to their advantage to reduce any unnecessary expense.

FUTURE TRENDS IN NOSOCOMIAL INFECTIONS: UNDERSTANDING SELECTIVITY AND SPECIFICITY IN MICROBIAL OPPORTUNISM

G.G. JACKSON

INTRODUCTION

A perspective of past experience

The principles involved and the principal types and causes of nosocomial infections occurring in recent years have been well recognized (1, 2). Past experience permits a valuable perspective for the future. Infections occurring in hospital patients reflect the epidemic waves of infection in the general population, especially those of respiratory diseases, but nosocomial infections differ by the occurrence of sporadic and endemic infections that are related to an altered host susceptibility to opportunistic microorganisms in the hospital setting. A wide variety of different host and hospital conditions are involved, and the resultant infections have greatly different biologic, clinical and economic consequences. Host specific attack rates are not known for most of the patient categories and prevalence rates of infection have been considered ranging from under 1 % (hip prosthesis) to 70 % in granulocytopenic, immunosuppressed patients.

Most preventive and therapeutic measures for nosocomial infections are judged without concommitant controls and are interpreted by historical experience. Such experience is variable according to the location and is influence by population density, age and disease related characteristics of the patients. The administration of antibiotics plays a minor role in determining the frequency of nosocomial infections, but is has a major effect on the nature of the causative bacterial strains. Intraoperative antibiotic prophylaxis reduces post operative infections in clean-contaminated and contaminated surgical procedures ; maximum environmental protection may further reduce the infection rate, but the percentage difference is small. Experience indicates that most prophylactic use and about one-half of therapeutic use of antibiotics fails to meet consensus standards. Preservation of the normal bowel flora and environmental protection have an additive effect in decreasing new colonization of the intestine. The prevalence of colonization with resistant strains of bacteria increases after 10 days of hospitalization. The spread of resistant strains can be minimized by barrier nursing and reduction of antibiotic usage. Multiple isolates of resistant bacteria and clusters of nosocomial infections in high-intensity care units are cause for alarm.

The outcome of treatment of hospital acquired infections is determined primarily by the underlying host disease. Successful treatment of sensitive strains is related to the site of infection, the pharmacokinetics and mechanisms of action of the drugs ; bacterial resistance tends to predict a poor clinical response. Evaluation of therapeutic measures depends on careful case stratification even among patients within a single disease category and the number of confounding variable requires caution in the interpretation of cause and effect relations.

Applications for the future

Future trends in the evaluation of nosocomial infections should be directed toward a better understanding of the selectivity and specificity of factors underlying opportunistic infections. Several areas of host parasite relations and the hospital environment hold promise for future efforts. They need to be examined individually and collectively as they apply to different aspects of nosocomial infections and selectively relate with different degrees of importance in specific situations. Some major areas are :

1) Recognizing microbial promoters of clinically important infections and of the interspecies transfer of microbial factors that are advantageous to their proliferation,

encroachment and virulence.

2) Relating reasons for certain kinds of infections to particular alteration in the immunologic host status that directly influence their frequency of acquisition, transmission and expression in disease.

3) Determining personnel directed practices, procedures, uses of equipment and drug administration that increase opportunities for infection ; and devising new methods to prevent or restrict microbial colonization, overgrowth, activation or invasion.

4) Developing recognition systems based on the nature of the patient's diseases and treatment that permit the earliest detection of pathologic changes in microbial flora or virulence, are predictive of untoward events and permit effective intervention for prevention or control of nosocomial infection.

5) Evaluating recommended activities for their cost effectiveness in lowering the frequency of nosocomial infections or preventing morbidity and mortality, noting those that are effective and those that are afforded for the improvement of professional standards.

SELECTIVITY AND SPECIFICITY IN OPPORTUNISTIC INFECTIONS

There are four categories of interacting factors that determine whether nosocomial infections occur, and if so, the kind of infection and its clinical course. Within each category are several features that affect the selectivity and specificity of opportunistic infections in the hospital setting. It is an increased understanding of the interplay and relevance of these individual features that is the challenge and promise of future observations and investigations of nosocomial infections. The promise of new information and understanding is great, because of the conditions imposed by microbial adaptation, the biologic effects of disease, the iatrogenic effects of patient care and the hospital as a social institution. The four categories and some of the features in each of them are outlined in Table 1.

Table 1.
SELECTIVITY AND SPECIFICITY IN NOSOCOMIAL INFECTIONS

EXOGENOUS (MICROBIAL) PROMOTERS

Bacterial conditioning for opportunism

- Gene transformation
- Plasmid transfer factors
- Inducible functions
- Mutation/Selection

Ecologic disruption and disproportionality

INTERVENING VECTORS

- Health care staff
- Equipment for diagnosis and therapy
- Biological products/Medicines
- Environment
  - Space/Person
  - Isolation facilities

INTERFACE PROMOTERS

- Creation of new portals of infection
- Bacterial adhesins
- Cytoreceptors
- Secretory and humoral reactants

INTERNAL (HOST) PROMOTERS

1) Endowment by age, sex, genes, experience, disease, drugs ;
2) Granulocytopenia/Poor granylocyte effectors ;
3) T-lymphocyte subset dyscoordination ;
4) Macrophage motivation/phagocytosis ;
5) Interrupted kinetic immunocommunications ;
6) Dysglobulinemia/Humoral cofactors.

MICROBIAL PROMOTERS OF INFECTION

In the recent past, aerobic gram-negative bacilli of the genus Enterobacteriacea or Pseudomonacea, many of which were formerly considered to be nonpathogenic have posed the greatest clinical problem. Formerly Staphylococci were the major problem. In the future as medical practices and the antimicrobial drugs are changed, there is no reason to believe that the present will be a permanent state with regard to the major causes of nosocomial infections. Recent observations have noted significant problems with methicillin-resistant

Staphylococcus aureus, Staphylococcus epidermidis, Bacteroides fragiles, coryneform bacteria, Mycobacterium cheloni, Legionella pneumoniae and other species not considered with much concern or even known by physicians until recently (1). Also, H. influenzae has demonstrated a new propensity for causing serious infections in adults. These events suggest a dynamic evolution in the species and properties of bacterial strains or conditions for the ecologic selection of unusual organisms. In part, these changes are effected by use of the antimicrobial durgs and evolve by basic microbiologic capabilities for change. Certain promoters of infection result in an increased number of organisms, a change in the local flora, or predominance of pathogenic species or strain.

Gene transformation

Changes in the constituitive gene of a bacterial strain can be accomplished in the laboratory by transduction. Similar events may occur in nature. To some extent the phenomenon of chromosomal alteration also can be accomplished by a phenomenon described as gene-hopping in which a constituitive gene is gained or lost from the cytoplasm by exchange with a plasmid component (3). Another provocative phenomenon observed in clindamycin resistant strains of B. fragilis is the inter-species transmissions of a non-plasmid borne resistance factor in which the conjugative transformation was promoted by sub-inhibitory concentrations of tetracycline (4). The observations suggest that transposons can be formed for the transfer of constituitive bacterial genes related to drug resistance independent of plasmid mediators and that antibiotic prescriptions can serve as a promoter.

Plasmid transfer factors

The role of plasmids in the transfer of bacterial resistance to antibiotics among strains of clinical importance has been well recognized. With the development of technology for identifying the molecular identity of particular plasmids and resistance factors by agarose gel electrophoreses and the endonuclease cleavage products of DNA, it has been possible to show that it is the plasmid transfer of the R-factor and not the genus or species identification of the infecting micro-organisms that is the important epidemiological event in endemics of nosocomial infection (5). Future considerations will need to observe the commonality of this marker in intrahospital infections and not just the carrier species of bacteria causing infection.

Inducible functions and mutational selections

Adaptive bacterial responses to the environment are numerous. Some of them are inducible. With the advent of cephalosporins that are resistant to the action of common microbial beta-lactamases, it has been observed that these compounds induce many strains to produce potent constituitive cephalosporinases and other beta-lactamases (6). This can be a dynamic function with a switch on/off responsiveness to the environmental milieu. Other observations have noted inducible tolerance of staphylococci and other species to the bacterial effects of antibiotics as an unstable form of resistance (7). These dynamic responses of bacteria to antibiotic exposure complement the selection of mutational resistance, when that occurs without loss of pathogenicity, in preserving an antibiotic resistant flora among hospital patients treated with antibiotics.

The selection of mutants that metabolically bypass a drug-induced blockade and other mechanisms such as the loss or alteration of drug receptors in the bacterial membrane or the diminution of autoenzymes that are target sites for drug actions favor these antimicrobial drug-resistant strains and promote their role in nosocomial infections of the predisposed patient. Together the various modes of bacterial response to local hospital practices insure the evolution of drug resistance and will serve to direct future changes in the etiologic nature of nosocomial infections within a particular hospital ward or unit. One can predict that the common types of nosocomial infections will continue to be caused by the prevalent species of bacteria that have acquired new capabilities for drug resistance through some of these mechanisms ; but also the increasing participation of unusual and pathogenically unrecognized species and strains can be expected.

Ecologic disruption and disproportionality

Bacterial interference among competitive elements is a dominant process in the establishment of the regional bacterial flora of the body, especially in the gastrointestinal and upper respiratory tracts and perhaps the skin. Elimination of the normal flora markedly increases the ease of colonization by other micro-organisms, including those with pathogenetic potential (8). Overgrowth of components of the normal flora increases the likelihood for extension of the growth into virgin areas with the production of disease. Drug resistance that reducesthe number of bacteria of potentially pathogenic species in the flora, while causing minimal disruption of other components, is a concept that is under investigation for the control of nosocomial infections in persons who are at unusually high risk of acquisition or extension of bacteria from colonized sites (9). The use of preserving rather than destroying adjunctive bacterial interference during antibiotic prophylaxis and treatment will have important future applications if the data from current investigations demonstrates a clinical advantage. As these new procedures permit longer term protection of highly susceptible persons, the relative importance of fungi and viruses, especially those that produce chronic or latent infections can be expected to emerge in importance as causes of acute nosocomial infections in these patients.

INTERVENING VECTORS

In the development of a large data base on the occurrence of nosocomial infections, the training of professional practicioners and the establishment of hospital requirements for infection control, it has been found that in most hospital situations the major component of preventable nosocomial infections is related to the intervening vectors surrounding the patient. In the hospital the interpersonal exchange of carrier strains is rapid and prevalent. The habits of the health care personnel are of paramount importance in reducing and containing endemic strains. The future requires of these personnel a continuing diligence, training and interest in this sector as the introduction of equipment for diagnosis and therapy is ever pervasive. Often little or no consideration is given to the use of a new appliance, test, procedure, or practice, for its effect as a portal or vector of nosocomial infections. It is necessary, therefore, to maintain a continuous awareness and assessment of these possibilities. Critical items in the environment are the amount of space per person and the availability of isolation facilities. It is in the monitoring and detection of intervening vectors of infection that the hospital epidemiologist and infection control practitioner have found the greatest opportunities and can continue to exercise an important influence in minimizing risks of nosocomial infection.

INTERFACE PROMOTERS

The interface between persons and microbes is altered by hospitalization itself, the disease states related to it, drugs administered, procedures used and especially surgical operations. Thus the nosocomial setting requires that a new equilibrium between host and microbes be reestablished frequently. The most overt and gross changes are those that create a new portal for bacterial entry. In these events, the role of an incision or insertion of a foreign body is self-evident. It must be expected that the use of surgery and artificial implants will continue to expand and the the occurrence or control of subsequent infections will be a major factor in establishing the limits and rate of expansion of such procedures.

Often the basis for the alteration of the host-microbe interface is more subtle. The bacterial flora of the oropharynx changes from gram-positive to gram-negative within hours after hospitalization and the initiation of intensive care (10). The change is unrelated to antibiotic administration and not clearly assignable to any recognized single specific event. The process is believed to reflect changes in substances at the interface between bacteria and host cells. For many infections, especially those originating in the respiratory or enteric tracts, the adherence of bacteria to specific cells of the mucosal lining is an essential step in the initiation of colonization, tissue invasion or toxicity. Certain bacterial products categorized as adhesins serve as specific ligands for binding bacteria to cells in a particular region (11). Sometimes they are present in the form of pili or fimbriae. Several classes of receptors on the surface of mucosal cells permit specific sugars (mannose, sialic acid or other), to serve as bacterial adhesins or ligands. Also important in the bacterial-cell interface responses are bacterial products such as some that chelate ferrous iron and can serve as selective local virulence factors. Fibronectin is a high molecular weight glyprotein found on the surface of many mucosal cells. It can serve as a receptor for staphylococci and an inhibitor to the attachment of Pseudomonas aeruginosa. Although their role is unresolved, these various bacterial products, adhesins and cytoreceptors appear to participate in the selectivity and specificity of infection that is a problem to be further worked out in future studies.

The mucosa of hollow organs that maintain a sterile environment such as the urinary bladder and perhaps the gall bladder and bronchioles exerts a bactericidal effect on adherent bacteria. Cytofusion and engulfment by pinocytosis are common processes occurring at the interface of bacteria with the mucosal surface. The accumulation of abnormal secretions, in volume or character, as is often caused by bedrest, disease, medications and procedures markedly alters the local conditions and adversely effects these controlling factors. When the secretions are exudative, immune complexes are formed with bacteria and bacterial products, complement is activated and leukocytes heighten the inflammatory manifestations of disease. Thus, there is a large number of still poorly understood specific and selective factors that operate at the level of the interface of mucosal cells and bacteria in establishing the local equilibrium with resultant sterility, colonization or disease. These relations are easily disturbed in the hospital environment and become determinants of acquisition of a new bacterial flora and nosocomial infection. The importance of increasing the knowledge in these areas is that the bacterial cell interface may be readily altered adversely or beneficially by many chemicals, subinhibitory concentrations of antibiotics and by vaccines. The identification of specific sites and antigens can provide the opportunity in the future for the development of drugs and antibody specifically directed at deterring bacterial adherence to cells.

INTERNAL (HOST) PROMOTERS

The immunologic and personal endowment that hospitalized patients bring with them is extremely diverse. The diseases and treatment as well as the setting create selective and specific provocative stress on some components of the host defense systems. What emerges is a rate and type of nosocomial infection. What underlies the facts is dysfunction of the host control measures owing to acquired, transiently affected or genetic immunologic deficiencies of individuals. Acquired infections themselves are increasingly being recognized as causing specific immunologic defects. As concepts and technologies are developed, an opportunity is provided to use observation of these stress conditions to understand more specifically the interlinked components of host responses that prevent or permit infections of certain types.

Patient groups for whom special characterization with regard to nosocomial infections is necessary are : newborns, especially if premature, post-surgical patients, those taking antiinflammatory drugs, asplenic persons and people hospitalized with recent or persistent viral or parasitic infections that have immunosuppressive effects ; two social customs, homosexual activity and drug abuse also produce infections with an immunosuppressive effect. The most overt altered host susceptibility occurs with iatrogenic immunosuppression of persons with neoplastic diseases and the recipients of organ homotransplants. Within each of these groups are subsets of patients and diseases with specific alterations that relate to their selective suceptibility to a particular type of nosocomial infection.

The occurrence of nosocomial infections provides an opportunity to observe in humans the operation of several specific immunologic functions which, for the most part, have been learned from animal experimentation. Some of the recognized segments of host immunity that are promotors of nosocomial infections are noted in Table 1. A continuing need is to make careful clinical and laboratory observations about the selectivity and sepcificity of the susceptibility of persons with particular disease states to various ubiquitous nosocomial micro-organisms. Already the general observations that relate humoral and phagocytic malfunctions to extracellular infections with some specificity for different kinds of micro-organisms ; and alterations in cell mediated immunity to intracellular bacterial infections, fungi and DNA viruses have been helpful as a descriptive basis for forming concepts.

A goal for the future is both better understanding of the processes involved, better determinations of the effect on the specificity of infection and the ability to devise selective remedies or reinforcement of specific responses that account for the particular host susceptibility that characterizes the different groups of patients. At the present time trends are being developed for granulocyte transfusions, autologous bone marrow implants, use of high titered immunoglobulins (with projections for exogenous production of monoclonal antibodies) preinduction immunization of patients to be given anticancer treatment and pretransplant immunologic conditioning of homograft recipients. Interferon to enhance natural killer cell activity, preparation of specific transfer factors and immuno enhancement by BCG (mycobacteria) are being investigated. Chemicals also are under study for their immunoregulatory effect on cell-mediated immunity. Among them are levamisol, cimetidine, muramyldipeptide, lithium, zinc and thymosin. Skilled observation and evaluation of these selective and specific regulatory functions is a great and exciting challenge for the future.

Although the identification of individual defects that are responsible for susceptibility to certain types of infection is the ideal, the different limbs of the immunologic defense system usually work in a multicellular and cascaded concert. An appreciation of this interdependence of the multifaceted aspects of host defense is as important to the understanding and prevention of nosocomial infections as is the desire to identify and understand the specific mechanisms that are involved. The care with which clinical observations are made will determine the rate of our improved understanding of these factors in patients.

SURVEILLANCE

Conscientious surveillance and tabulation of nosocomial infections can serve as a quality control within a hospital or unit, permit early recognition of emerging problems, show the changing virulence and/or prevalence of a particular bacterial strain, give a focus for directed efforts toward infection control and sometimes serve as an index of the effect of new recommendations, Some surveillance to sustain these recognized benefits and provide a local educational presence have been generally established and sometimes mandated by law. There are two aspects of surveillance to be considered.
a) Detection of clinical infections by inspection of the patient and/or hospital record for the determination of prevalence rates of infection at different sites among patients in various units of the hospital. In the past this type of effort has uncovered the bulk of the common preventable infections which involve mainly the urinary tract, respiratory tract, wounds or skin. There is a limit to what can be done

in the prevention of infections by such surveillance. When stable and acceptable rates are observed, different forms of monitoring can be used and the effort switched to directed investigations. b) Surveillance of bacterial cultures submitted to the hospital laboratory. With increasing computerization of laboratory results it will be relatively easier in the future to develop a system of "alarm reports". These may identify a noticeable increase in the number of cultures submitted, a clustering of positive results, the emergence of a certain strain or the development of new bacterial resistance to one or more antibiotics. Even without computerization the occurrence of urinary tract infections, the most common type of nosocomial infection can be used as an index of prevalence and the results of positive wound or blood cultures used as a monitor for the detection of invasive bacterial strains (12). The sensitivity of the alarm reports can be set in each hospital to use the personnel most efficiently in the investigation of emerging risks.

PREDICTIVE CULTURES

Most surveillance is of value in making retrospective interpretations. It can have extended value by improving procedures and conditions which reduce the risk of patient acquisition of nosocomial infection on a statistical basis, although this can be difficult to prove. Risk of nosocomial infection is an individual matter that is determined by the circumstances of a particular patient. Research protocols have begun to develop data on the predictive value of results of cultures in high risk neutropenic and/or immunosuppressed patients (13). Among such persons the initial presence of gram-negative bacilli in the oropharynx was observed to be associated with an increase of up to 20 % in the number of patient days with respiratory infection (from 13 % to 33 % of the days) and if the isolate of gram-negative bacilli was acquired in the hospital the percentage of days with respiratory infection increased from 13 % to 46 % (14). Similar data have been obtained with regard to the risk of bacteremia (15) and are shown in Table 2. A noteworthy observation is that intestinal colonization with Ps. aeruginosa in the hospital was predictive of subsequent bacteremia with a 40 % likelihood.

Table 2.

PREDICTIVE VALUE OF TWICE WEEKLY CULTURES IN 128 PATIENTS WITH NONLYMPHOCYTIC LEUKEMIA 1969-1976

	Number with Bacteremia / Number Colonized			
	Present on admission		Aquired in hospital	
Pseudomonas aeruginosa	7/25	(28 %)	16/41	(40 %)
E. coli	15/104	(14 %)	3/33	(9 %)
Klebsiella species (incl. pneumoniae)	15/68	(22 %)	6/51	(12 %)
Proteus species	2/53	(4 %)	1/40	(3 %)
Enterobacter cloacae	0/30	(0)	0/38	(0)

Adapted from reference 15

Other data suggest predictive interpretation of fungal cultures for the development of systemic fungal disease (16). A negative culture for Candida albicans in the respiratory secretions, urine or stool was reliable evidence against the development of systemic candidiasis. A positive culture had no significant predictive merit. Negative cultures for aspergillus were not a reliable indicator to exclude the infection. In contrast to C. albicans, a positive culture for C. tropicalis was associated with the development of systemic candidiasis in 60 % of the observations.

Although routine predictive culturing is not presently recommended, these are the kinds of data that future surveillance will want to provide as the observations on specificity and selectivity of certain species become clearly related to predictable events.

COST EFFECTIVENESS

Nosocomial infections collectively represent a modern day epidemic of microbial diseases. Much has been accomplished in the recognition of this fact and the detection of preventable causes of infection. The cost of such infections in terms of illnes, loss of life and additional expense to the person and society are very large. The remaining preventable component of some types of infection is limited within the confines of accepted practices and treatment and requires continous redefinition. Although we would like to assume that all nosocomial infections are preventable, the provisions required for the further reduction can be very expensive. It is a characteristic of modern medical capability to be able theoretically to do more than can be afforded with a reasonable distribution of fiscal resources. A major challenge for the future is to set priorities in the allocation of time, funds, developmental procedures and research to maintain the lowest possible occurrence of nosocomial infection, the most effective management of those that occur and to increase knowledge pertaining to the basic biology of opportunistic infections.

REFERENCES

1. Second international conference on nosocomial infections, R.E. Dixon, Ed. 1981. Am. J. Med. 70 : Part I : 379, Part II : 631, Part III : 899.
2. Bennett, J.V., Brachman, P.S., Editors. 1980. Hospital Infections, Little, Brown and Co. Boston, Mass.
3. Gold Spring Harbor Symp. Quant. Biol. 1981 : 45, Movable genetic elements pp. 445.
4. Tally, F., Jacobs, N. 1982. Multicenter survey of Bacteroides susceptibility in the U.S. Abstracts, Ann. Mtg. ASM A-66.
5. Rubens, C.E., Farrar, W.E. Jr., McGee, Z.A., Schaffner, W. 1981. Evolution of plasmid mediating resistance to multiple antimicrobial agents during a prolonged epidemic of nosocomial infections. J. Inf. Dis. 143 : 170.
6. Sanders, C.C., Moellering, R.C. Jr., Martin, R.R. 1982. Resistance to cephamondole : A collaborative study of emerging clinical problems. J. Inf. Dis. 145 : 118.
7. Nelson, R.E., Washington, J.A. 1981. Paradoxic and tolerant effects of moxalactam on Staphylococcus aureus. J. Inf. Dis. 144 : 178.

8. Thijn, H.A., Waaij, D. van der. 1979. The effect of three frequently applied antibiotics on the colonization resistance of the digestive tract of mice. J. Hyg. Camb. 82 : 397.
9. Guiot, H.F.L., Meer, J.W.M. van der, Furth, R. van. 1981. Selective antimicrobial modulation of microbial human flora : Infection prevention in patients with decreased host defense mechanisms by selective elimination of potentially pathogenic bacteria. J. Inf. Dis. 143 : 644.
10. Johanson, W.G., Pierce, A.K., Sanford, J.P., Thomas, G.D. 1972. Nosocomial respiratory infections with gram-negative bacilli. The significance of colonization of the respiratory tract. Ann. Int. Med. 77 : 701.
11. Beachey, E.H. 1981. Bacterial adherence : Adhesin receptor interactions mediating the attachment of bacteria to mucosal surfaces. J. Inf. Dis. 143 : 325.
12. Jackson, G.G. 1978. The role of the laboratory in providing microbiological data. In : Proven and Unproven Methods in Hospital Infection Control, F. Daschner, Ed. Verlag, N.Y.
13. Schimpff, S.C. 1981. Surveillance cultures. J. Inf. Dis. 144 : 81.
14. Kurrle, E., Bhaduri, S., Krieger, W., et al. 1981. Risk factors for infections of the oropharynx and respiratory tract in patients with acute leukemia. J. Inf. Dis. 144 : 128.
15. Newman, K.A., Schimpff, S.C., Young, V.M., Weirnik, P.H. 1981. Lessons learned from surveillance cultures in patients with acute nonlymphocytic leukemia : usefulness for epidemiologic, preventive and therapeutic research. Am. J. Med. 70 : 423.
16. Sandford, G.R., Merz, W.G., Wingard, J.R., et al. 1980. The value of fungal surveillance cultures as predictors of systemic fungal infections. J. Inf. Dis. 142 : 503.

GPSR Compliance
The European Union's (EU) General Product Safety Regulation (GPSR) is a set of rules that requires consumer products to be safe and our obligations to ensure this.

If you have any concerns about our products, you can contact us on

ProductSafety@springernature.com

In case Publisher is established outside the EU, the EU authorized representative is:

Springer Nature Customer Service Center GmbH
Europaplatz 3
69115 Heidelberg, Germany

www.ingramcontent.com/pod-product-compliance
Ingram Content Group UK Ltd.
Pitfield, Milton Keynes, MK11 3LW, UK
UKHW020248290926
15470UKWH00002B/808
9789024727544